A Medical Companion to Dickens's Fiction

European University Studies

Europäische Hochschulschriften
Publications Universitaires Européennes

Series XIV
Anglo-Saxon Language and Literature

Reihe XIV Série XIV
Angelsächsische Sprache und Literatur
Langue et littérature anglo-saxonnes

Vol./Bd. 417

PETER LANG
Frankfurt am Main · Berlin · Bern · Bruxelles · New York · Oxford · Wien

Joanne Eysell

A Medical Companion to Dickens's Fiction

PETER LANG
Europäischer Verlag der Wissenschaften

Bibliographic Information published by Die Deutsche Bibliothek
Die Deutsche Bibliothek lists this publication in the Deutsche Nationalbibliografie; detailed bibliographic data is available in the internet at <http://dnb.ddb.de>.

ISSN 0721-3387
ISBN 3-631-54123-6
US-ISBN 0-8204-7743-5

www.peterlang.de

In memory of my grandfather

Dr Charles Edwin Ames

Preface and Acknowledgements

The impetus to writing this thesis was given in the number of articles which have appeared - and continue to appear - in medical journals from time to time about Dickens or his characters.

None of this dissertation has been previously published, but an overview of the material was presented, with particular discussion of smallpox in *Bleak House* and the postulated use of leukaemia in *Dombey and Son,* in March 2000 to the Section of Medical History of the North Staffordshire Medical Institute, Stoke-on-Trent.

The following editions and abbreviations have been used for primary sources. Page numbers of quotations from Dickens's works are given in parentheses at the end of the quotation, preceded by these abbreviations.

(PP) *Pickwick Papers.* Oxford World's Classics, 1988.
James Kinsley, ed.
(OT) *Oliver Twist.* Oxford, Clarendon Press, 1974.
Kathleen Tillotson, ed.
(NN) *Nicholas Nickleby.* Oxford, Oxford University Press, 1982.
(OCS) *The Old Curiosity Shop.* Oxford, Clarendon Press, 1997.
Elizabeth Brennan, ed.
(BR) *Barnaby Rudge.* London, Penguin, 1986. Gordon Spence, ed.
(MC) *Martin Chuzzlewit.* Oxford, Clarendon Press, 1982.
Margaret Cardwell, ed.
(DS) *Dombey and Son.* Oxford World's Classics, 1996.
Alan Horsman, ed.
(DC) *David Copperfield.* Oxford, Clarendon Press, 1981.
Nina Burgess, ed.
(BH) *Bleak House.* London. Penguin, 1994.
(HT) *Hard Times.* London. Penguin, 1983. David Craig, ed.
(LD) *Little Dorrit.* Oxford, Clarendon Press, 1979.
Harvey Peter Sucksmith, ed.
(TTC) *A Tale of Two Cities.* London, Penguin, 1988.
George Woodcock, ed.
(GE) *Great Expectations.* New York, Norton, 1999.
Edgar Rosenberg, ed.
(OMF) *Our Mutual Friend.* London, Penguin, 1987. Stephen Gill, ed.
(ED) *Mystery of Edwin Drood.* Oxford, Clarendon Press, 1972.
Margaret Cardwell, ed.
The Christmas Books, London, Penguin, reprint 1984. Michael Slater, ed. "A Christmas Carol" and "The Chimes"

(SB)	*Sketches by Boz* in *Dickens' Journalism*, 1. London, Phoenix. Michael Slater, ed.
(UT)	*Uncommercial Traveller* in *Dickens' Journalism*, 4. London, Dent. Michael Slater, ed.
(AN)	*American Notes*. London. Penguin, 1987. John Whitley and Arnold Goldman, eds.
(Letters)	*Letters of Charles Dickens*. Oxford. The Pilgrim Edition. Madeline House, et al. eds.
(Speeches)	*The Speeches of Charles Dickens*. A Complete Edition. Hemel Hempstead, Harvester Wheatsheaf. K.J. Fielding, ed.
(HW)	*Household Words*. London, Bradbury and Evans.
(AYR)	*All the Year Round*. London, Chapman and Hall.
(Marigold)	"Dr Marigold's Prescriptions". New York, The New York Publishing Company

Illustrations are included with kind permission of the following:

Originals from Dickens's works	The Dickens Museum, London
The Empty Chair	The Dickens Museum, London
Henry VIII and the Barber Surgeons	Worshipful Society of Barbers
The Doctor	Tate Gallery

My thanks are expressed to a number of people who have given so much support and encouragement: my two supervisors, Prof. Dennis Walder of the Open University, in literature and Prof. Ulrich Tröhler of the University of Freiburg, in medical history; Dr David Parker, Dr John Cosnett and Dr Anthony Carter, David Dickens, Michael Fife, Peter Schmidt, Michael Bauer, my proofreaders Anita Zelasny and Dr Susanne Keil, and last but by no means least, my husband Rolf.

TABLE OF CONTENTS

List of Illustrations

INTRODUCTION

Generations of readers have read and reread Dickens's novels, savouring his genius for description and characterization. The number, variety and quality of medical descriptions presented appear, however, to have gone largely unnoticed. Certainly, the conspicuous cases involving death, like Smike or Little Nell, or the near demise of Tiny Tim and Esther Summerson are known, but recognition seldom goes beyond these. Articles in medical journals tend to focus on a single condition and retrospective diagnosis, while the general public almost entirely overlooks the medical argument.[1]

In approaching this topic, the following questions for investigation have crystallized out of the materials available: First, how does Dickens appear to view medical practitioners? Second, which identifiable diseases are to be found in Dickens's fiction? Third, which diseases does Dickens use in prominent focus in his works? Fourth, what specific remedies does Dickens describe? And last, what role do public health issues, popular (orthodox and unorthodox) medical movements or superstitions play? The present *Companion* illuminates the medical environment in which Dickens was writing and provides a contextualised reference guide to the diseases, morbid states and remedies to be found in his fiction.

As Umberto Eco said in an essay published in 1997:

> Anyone who begins to examine something has first at least formulated the beginning of a thought process which induces him to follow one hypothesis rather than another.[2]

The hypothesis which I have been 'induced to follow' is based on a statement by the mid-twentieth century physician Lord Brain, that Dickens was an astute observer of physical morbid states. [3] This motivated the research in medical literature from Dickens's day to the present behind my thesis. My intent is a fairly comprehensive, though not exhaustive, summary of available articles along with a review of the medical episodes, morbid states and remedies in their Dickensian and contemporary-medical setting. Thus far, science *per se* has been increasingly examined in literary criticism, though as Sally Shuttleworth points out, "Victorian science was not . . . a unified body of knowledge, but rather a diffuse collection of disciplines . . .[4] Medicine is one such discipline, but we must also be aware that it was nowhere near as "scientific" as it was to become in the late nineteenth and even more in the twentieth century. One other major factor we must keep in mind is that, for Dickens, medicine was still the healing *art* of earlier times. He was certainly aware of advances in medicine, but this is seldom reflected in his fiction. Examination of Dickens's medical episodes from a literary point of view reveals his genius for word play, interweaving for example physical blindness and metaphorical blindness in *Barnaby Rudge*.[5] Examination of Dickens's fiction from a *medical-historical* point of view brings the realization that his clinical descriptions were not solely a matter of aesthetics; he chose frequently to include details where he could have been vague – and occasionally chose to be vague in order to strengthen an effect. The facet of Dickens's work examined here is the *quality* of his medical descriptions *per se*. That is, medical realism as observed and depicted by Dickens is the focus, rather than the literary construct. This is not to say that medicine and literature are – or even could be - completely divorced in this dissertation. Dickens worked medical realism into literary convention, using for example what Susan Sontag, in her *Illness as Metaphor,* calls the "mythology" of tuberculosis - the images associated with this disease in the lay mind. I will return to some of her insights in Chapter 5, but for the most part, my aim is summarized in Sontag's statement:

> My point is that illness is *not* a metaphor, and that the most truthful way of regarding illness . . . is the one most purified of . . . metaphoric thinking.[6]

What I want to examine here is *which* diseases and health topics Dickens described and *how* he did so, rather than which social ills – for social ills were usually the target – Dickens was attacking metaphorically. Dickens's involvement in the amelioration of such ills has been extensively documented; this dissertation provides information on the *medical* environment in which Dickens's novels were written as a supplement to the increasingly investigated political, social, colonial and reform environments.

For these purposes, it is not necessary to reiterate here all the developments in literary criticism of Dickens's works. A brief but very useful summary of the various schools of thought, beginning with G.H. Lewes and George Eliot through Freudian, to Foucauldian and feminist readings of the late twentieth century is given, for example, in Lyn Pykett's *Charles Dickens*.[7] More specifically germane to my discussion, M. Anne Crowther's article in the *Oxford Reader's Companion to Dickens*[8] presents a general discussion of the current *literary*-critical view of "health, illness, and disability" in Dickens's works, highlighting in particular the high mortality rates in the nineteenth century and their effects on the literature of the age. Crowther points out that Dickens is "rarely specific on the causes of non-accidental death in his fiction,"[9] which is correct if one understands being "specific" in the sense of naming the cause. Based on the details in Dickens's descriptions, physicians have found it fascinating to identify not only the cause of death but non-fatal morbid states which Dickens chose to include in his works. Thus, while Crowther rightly states that social neglect and poverty are behind the plight of such characters as Jo, Tiny Tim and Jenny Wren, the medical profession sets aside the literary, socio-critical importance of the description and attempts to arrive at a diagnosis.

This does not imply that the profession ignores the metaphorical use or negates its importance, but emphasises Dickens's powers of observation. It also emphasises the degree to which Dickens's characters still "live" more than a century after their creation.

This dissertation is intended as a companion or guide to aid examination of specifically *medical* episodes and descriptions. It provides a summary of and information about physical diseases as well as specific remedies described by Dickens in his novels and sketches. Information to facilitate examination of the neglected historical context is provided by demonstrating Dickens's awareness of medicine and medical practice in his time. Medical literature is reviewed to illustrate the reception of his works by the profession. A wide variety of medical and hospital journals has been consulted and relevant articles collected and made easily searchable for non-medical readers. Thus, this dissertation provides a basis for literary examination of medical discourse comparable to publications available on the works of Flaubert, Balzac and Eliot.[10]

Psychosomatic medicine is not included in this review, despite the awareness of emotional factors in disease among nineteenth-century practitioners. This is not to say that Dickens was unaware of or not interested in both the factors and contemporary discussions thereof. His descriptions of the illnesses of Madeline Bray, Nell's grandfather and Pip are cases in point. My viewpoint here, however, is that of the initial examiner in the early stages of diagnosis. Paralleling today's medical practice of first examining a patient physically then recommending psychotherapy if appropriate, this thesis identifies and discusses descriptions of physical disease; psychosomatics should be the topic of a separate examination.

Medical Realism

According to Shuttleworth, "realism is a term invoked to offer an air of critical plausibility to the critic's own subjective projections onto the text."[11] Ascribing what, for the purposes of this dissertation, I wish to call "medical realism" (as opposed to literary realism) to Dickens's works involves issues of "diagnosing" fictitious characters. One approach is *historical interpretation*, based on examination of medical texts available in Dickens's day. Another approach is *retrospective diagnosis*, which requires interpretation of descriptions on the basis of modern knowledge.[12] Many of the Dickens-related articles in medical publications are based on this latter approach and reveal several morbid states which Dickens described with considerable accuracy before their inclusion in medical literature. In reviewing Dickens's descriptions, I have relied on the interpretations by medical professionals and, aware of the liabilities of retrospective diagnoses,[13] subjected these to historical examination. I thereby arrived at interpretations which in some cases differ from the published opinion (which is frequently inconsistent within itself).

The question arises about Dickens's sources beyond his own keen powers of observation. Unfortunately, any answer must remain speculative. There were several medical books in Dickens's library[14] as potential sources. We know that there were several doctors among his friends and acquaintances and that he was acquainted with Thomas Wakley, the founder of the reform-oriented medical journal *The Lancet*. He supported several projects of committees established by *The Lancet* and may well have read the journal. Dickens also makes mention in *Little Dorrit* of "the most widely-read nonreligious book in the English language during the half century following its Edinburgh publication in 1769"[15] – that is, William Buchan's *Domestic Medicine, or a Treatise on the Prevention and Cure of Diseases by Regime and Simple Medicine*. The 1828 edition, which Dickens would plausibly have known, contains several articles which might have been of help to him. But again, this is speculation.

The topics examined in this dissertation can be grouped into the following categories: medical personnel, specific morbid states, public health issues (these two overlap somewhat) and folk medicine/superstitions.

Medical Personnel

Addressing the broad spectrum of topics as outlined above, I have chosen to begin with a review of the medical practitioners created by Dickens. Here, we begin to see the development of Dickens's attitude toward the profession and also find evidence of his awareness of the structures and politics involved.

About 50 medical men appear in Dickens's works.[16] (Gender was not a question in the nineteenth century; while not illegal, it was very rare for women to practice medicine in Britain at the time.) The more prominent of these characters were the focus of medical reception of Dickens's works up to about 1955. After that time, the focus changed toward the medical topics in his works. Again, my viewpoint in this discussion is not that of the literary critic: the doctor's function within the plot is of less interest here than Dickens's description of the man's training and activities.

Specific morbid states

There are many specific physical morbid states described by Dickens which do not necessarily play a major part in the plot or affect the message of the work. Chapter 2 presents an overview of these states, beginning with the Pickwick Syndrome because of its obvious relationship to the first novel. Since these states are not interrelated and are to be found scattered throughout Dickens's fiction, I have simply arranged the rest in alphabetical order for the reader's convenience, with repeated descriptions then in chronological order of the works. A glossary of the medical terms used is provided in Appendix 2.

Dickens – like most Victorian novelists – usually did not name the disease he had in mind. My discussion is therefore based on retrospective diagnoses reported in medical journals of the twentieth and twenty-first centuries and tested against medical sources of the nineteenth. The range extends from diseases afflicting the individual character to diseases afflicting large segments of the population. In both categories there are descriptions which are essential to the particular novel, but also descriptions which now seem entirely secondary. The fascinating point is that the descriptions are equally realistic, regardless of their metaphorical importance in the novel. Dickens's major pictures of morbid states differ from his minor clinical descriptions more in the obviousness of their purpose and repetition in the novels than in their accuracy of detail.

Unlike the morbid states comprising Chapter 2, there are four diseases or disorders which are used in prominent focus in Dickens's works. I have dedicated a separate chapter to each of these: epilepsy, stroke, tuberculosis and smallpox. Reading from a medical-historical point of view brings out features of these cases which highlight Dickens's grasp of the morbid state and illustrate that his use includes more than just the customary tropes. New insight thus obtained is the political thrust found for epilepsy and smallpox. Examination of the cause of stroke in Dickens's fiction reveals a symbolic retributive use which has not been identified in earlier discussions. While some attention is paid in these chapters to the literary/metaphorical use, the main focus remains on Dickens's medical description and its realism. The arrangement of the chapters leads from the individual sufferer to society at large: epilepsy and stroke are non-contagious and afflict individual sufferers, while tuberculosis and smallpox were rampant during the nineteenth century. This leads into a discussion in Chapter 7 of general public health issues.[17]

Public health issues

Dickens's descriptions of public health issues which were under legislation or discussed in the medical press are reviewed from the Dickens-contemporary medical perspective. Laymen might object to calling some of these issues "medical" (there is no patient who can be diagnosed and treated). Indeed, the public health movement in the nineteenth century was largely hampered in its early phase by arguments between economists like Chadwick and the medical profession about the knowledge most needed to solve the problems. Gradually, clinical medicine took precedence over economics and public health is seen now as a separate specialty within health care – but increasingly returning to control by the economists. Dickens voiced concern about these issues and expended considerable energy to help bring about their amelioration. Chapter 7 illustrates the now nearly-forgotten topicality of this aspect of Dickens's novels and sketches.

Folk Medicine and Superstition

Dickens, as a popular novelist, would perhaps be expected to make use of folk medicine. This is found to be true. Review of Dickens's correspondence reveals which of these remedies were used in his family, and comparison with Dickens-contemporary medical literature identifies which were approved by the medical profession.

Dickens makes little use of superstition; the most prominent case is, of course, spontaneous human combustion. It can be seen, however, that this topic was included in texts on medical jurisprudence (where it still is found), and serious texts on the subject were written late in the twentieth century, bringing its classification as "superstition" into question. Here, again, literary criticism has addressed the metaphoric use of the phenomenon nearly to the exclusion of the medical discussion. The aim here is not to reiterate known articles, but to present the less-known medical sources.

Conclusions

Dickens's interest in the unusual led him to observe not only the social details for which he is so justly famous, but also details of nineteenth-century medicine. In this thesis, I highlight Dickens's medical descriptions and place them in relation to the medical environment in which the novels were written. This provides a new and fascinating vantage point from which to examine the works as an integral part of the Victorian Age. Although some morbid states appear to have been described simply because Dickens observed them, the topicality of several of the diseases and socio-medical issues addressed by Dickens has been hitherto overlooked or obscured by time. Noteworthy in the writings of a medical layman, descriptions of the same disease in different novels are not merely repeated, but various aspects of the disease are highlighted, making the use unique to that novel. Perhaps unknown outside the medical community, comparison of Dickens's writings with medical texts of his day reveals that his descriptions preceded medical publication in several instances. This presentation locates the medical episodes within the vastness of Dickens's fiction to facilitate investigation of questions concerning changing metaphors over time, the impact of disease prevalence on literature, the use of language in describing illness and other related topics.

Looking at this aspect of Dickens's works will help to fill in one of the blanks remaining in our understanding of his genius for observation and description. This talent has been noticed by the medical profession in the past, but the scope and width of his observations in this field seem not to have been given sufficient publicity and credit. By placing Dickens's works within the context of nineteenth-century medicine, this thesis aims to make another aspect of his work available for general readers as well as for specialist researchers.

---

[1] See medical journal articles in the bibliography.
[2] Eco (2000); 44: my translation from a translation by Burkart Kroebar.
[3] Brain (1955), 136.
[4] Shuttleworth (1984), X.
[5] See below, page 79.
[6] Sontag (1979), 3.
[7] Pykett (2002).
[8] Schlicke (1999), 266-68. Reference is made to other articles in the volume where appropriate.
[9] Ibid, 267.
[10] See for example Rothfield (1999), *Vital Signs.*
[11] Shuttleworth (1984) 489.
[12] For a discussion of these methods and related problems, see Leven in Paul and Schlich (1998), 153-185.
[13] Peter Stanley reminds his readers that "Retrospective and speculative diagnosis is enjoyable but hazardous, and correction encourages unproductive condescension." (Stanley (2003), 52).
[14] See list in Appendix 3.
[15] Furst (1998), 30.
[16] A complete list is found in Appendix 1.
[17] See Appendix 4 for articles in *Household Words* and *All the Year Round*, and his speeches.

CHAPTER 1: Dickens's Medical Practitioners

The doctor and his literary role are less conspicuous in Dickens's works than medicine and disease, in which Dickens's observations and descriptions are extremely perspicacious. Since, however, medicine and medical episodes cannot be entirely divorced from the practitioners, I will start my study with those. This also reflects the situation for more than half a century after Dickens's death, when articles in medical journals mostly concentrated on the doctors and their possible models.

It can be expected of a great observer like Dickens that his portrayal of the medical profession will give us some insight into conditions prevailing in the nineteenth century. Certainly, we must allow for satire, for caricature and perhaps some not very thinly-veiled criticism. It cannot be expected that Dickens would hold back in describing the medical profession, any more than he did with the law, for instance. And indeed this is the case. While the characters might show "less seriousness of purpose than Lydgate in *Middlemarch*," they are nevertheless considered to be "deeply interesting as types."[1] In many of Dickens's books, someone is hurt or becomes ill and requires medical attendance, which is duly provided by an anonymous person. In other works, the doctor's role is more prominent and he takes part in dialogue. Apart from Allan Woodcourt in *Bleak House*, however, the doctor hardly attains the prominence of lawyers in Dickens's fiction. Even Woodcourt is not as important to the action of the novel as the several lawyers. Consistent with the expected frequency of encounter in most people's lives, there are more doctors than lawyers (the counts are about 50:20), but there is no single doctor in any of the novels who has the importance in the story of Mr Wickfield, Betsey Trotwood's solicitor, and his clerk, Uriah Heep, who far overshadow Mr Chillip in *David Copperfield.* The two lawyers, Stryver and Carton, who are involved in Charles Darney's trial for espionage in *A Tale of Two Cities*, stand out more, professionally, than Dr Manette, even though the doctor is the key figure and the novel was almost entitled *The Doctor of Beauvais*. And in the last of Dickens's completed novels, *Our Mutual Friend*, two of the main characters, Mortimer Lightwood and Eugene Wrayburn, are lawyers, while there is no named doctor at all. But more importantly, while lawyers are almost always negatively represented, medical men, even where criticized, are viewed more positively. Philip Collins sees this as a general rule and not Dickens-specific:

> The doctor has the advantage over the solicitor, in popular fiction, that lawyers are traditionally regarded with suspicion, hatred or derision, where doctors – unless they are manifestly quacks – are generally respected.[2]

Examination of the more than 50 characters pertinent to this study would appear to necessitate a novel-by-novel summary for orientation, but most of the figures do not warrant such attention. The medical figures discussed in this study are those who were singled out for attention among medical readers over the years. It is seen that in portraying medical practitioners, as in all other aspects of his writing, Dickens draws on literature and life, demonstrably weaving what he observed with what he had read, fact with fiction, reality with fantasy and past with present.

Historical overview

A brief introduction to the history of medical training and its development in Victorian Britain will help our understanding of why Dickens portrayed medical figures as he did.

Traditionally, the medical profession in Britain was separated into three orders: physicians, surgeons and apothecaries. Of these, only the physician was required to have university training. Fellowship in the oldest medical corporation - the Royal College of Physicians, chartered in 1518 by Henry VIII - was restricted to graduates of Oxford and Cambridge. While Scottish universities provided better practical medical education than either Oxford or Cambridge, these latter gave students "an education in morals and manners that made them fit candidates for the Fellowship (F.R.C.P.)." [3] Lesser lights could be licensed (L.R.C.P.) to practice medicine; those wishing to practice in London were, in fact, required to be licensed, whereas licensing was optional for practitioners in rural areas.

Surgery, by contrast, was "skilled manual labour." [4] Surgeons were originally part of the Guild of Barbers and trained by apprenticeship. Until 1540, there were two bodies: the Barbers Company, chartered in 1462, and the Fellowship of Surgeons. Members of the former who practiced surgery were known as "barber-surgeons" while the members of the latter practiced only surgery. In 1540, an Act of Parliament was passed - only applicable to London and the environs in a one-mile circumference - separating the barbers from the surgeons. This measure prohibited barbers from surgical practice (excepting dental extractions) and surgeons from barbering, with the intention of reducing the spread of infectious diseases. The new body formed was called "The Worshipful Company of Barbers and Surgeons of London". Possibly in commemoration of this, Holbein painted "Henry VIII and the Barber Surgeons".

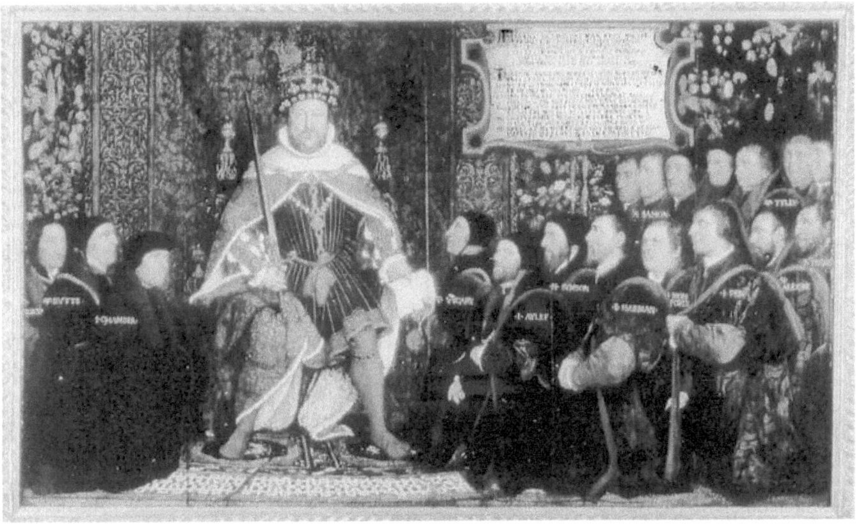

Fig. 1: Holbein: "Henry VIII and the Barber Surgeons." The Worshipful Society of Barbers.

Contributing further to the confusion, the Latin text shown in the painting calls the barbers "medici" or physicians. The Royal College of Surgeons was not chartered until 1800, with a new charter in 1843 defining the functions of the surgeon and membership in the college.

Apothecaries, the third group to practice medicine, were originally grocers who mixed and dispensed remedies. This is reflected in *Martin Chuzzlewit:* "Now, there being no medical practitioner actually resident in the village, but a poor apothecary who was also a grocer and general dealer..." (*MC,* 26) and again in *Dombey and Son*: after the collapse of the House, Towlinson, the footman, and Annie, the maid, resolve "to take one another for better, for worse, and to settle in Oxford Market in the general green grocery and herb and leech line." (*DS,* 872) It was apothecaries rather than physicians or surgeons who were the first general practitioners,[5] often asked for advice before - or instead of - consulting the doctor, who had to be paid. They gained legal sanction in the early eighteenth century to prescribe medications, were allowed, however, only to charge for the medications they sold and not for advice given.[6] The Apothecaries Act of 1815 made it legal for them to practice medicine on completion of an apprenticeship.

The title "doctor" was restricted to men with university training in medicine, that is, the physicians. Surgeons were addressed as "Mr" but in speaking of the profession, it was common to use the word "doctor" for any practitioner. The general public did not make the distinction and the medical profession itself discussed eliminating the difference in title. The *British Medical Journal* of September 25, 1869 asked: "Is it well that the distinction between "doctor" and "surgeon" should be any longer maintained?" The writer pointed out that there was no longer any difference in the practice, education or fees charged.

The division persists – as does the confusion, especially for non-British readers. Professor Edgar Rosenberg, editor of the Norton Critical Edition of *Great Expectations* (1999), includes a footnote to explain a comment that Jaggers "washed his clients off, as if he were a surgeon or a dentist." Rosenberg writes: "In England the term surgeon refers to all physicians; the surgery is the examination room."[7] This was not correct at the time Dickens was writing, nor is it entirely accurate now.

The doctor in fiction

Illness has always held a certain fascination for observers both in real life and in fiction. Thinking of Victorian fiction, we perhaps envision melodrama and pathos, to which death-bed scenes lend themselves particularly well. One then assumes a doctor in attendance; caring but basically – given the state of Victorian medicine - helpless. Many of the now-eradicated diseases were rampant and untreatable a century ago. The painting "The Doctor" by Sir Luke Fildes (1891) reflects this: the doctor sits, simply watching, by the bed of his young patient.

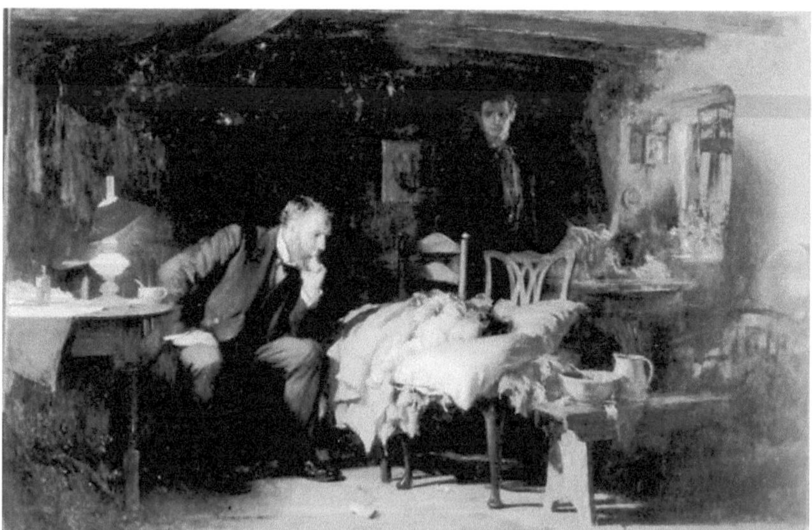

Fig. 2: Fildes: "The Doctor." The Tate Gallery.

There have been many and sometimes rapid changes both during and since Victorian times,[8] and having had instilled since the early twentieth century belief in the doctor as demigod, practically infallible and omniscient, today's lay readers may expect doctors in fiction to reflect that belief. The question is, does Dickens support this medical self-aggrandizement? What impression do we get of his view of medicine and the medical profession?

Two essays would appear to promise useful guidelines for the interpretation of doctors' roles in Dickens's fiction from a lay-literary point of view: Q.D. Leavis's "The Symbolic Function of the Doctor in Victorian Novels," published as an appendix to her essay "Bleak House. A Chancery World"[9] and Philip Collins's "Physicians in Victorian Fiction".[10] As the titles indicate, there are similarities in these essays and they do provide a literary reading mode which might serve as a basis for study. For the medical reading mode, we turn to articles published in medical and hospital journals over the years.

The nineteenth century brought enormous changes in many fields. Medicine was not exempt. New theories questioned or confirmed earlier "facts", medicine began its development from an art into modern medical science, and the doctor became more of a healer, with increasingly sophisticated means of diagnosis and treatment at his disposal. As Leavis points out, it was only with the social and medical changes in the nineteenth century that the fictional role of the doctor became that of a "modern" practitioner. "Thus," she writes, "he became an evident symbol and available as such to the novelist as a central character instead of a stock background filler."[11] Considering Dickens's doctors, however, one may question the degree to which they can be considered symbolic. Nor, as we will see, are very many of Dickens's doctors "central characters." Even Allan Woodcourt in *Bleak House,* whom Leavis mentions in this regard, is absent from England for much of the narrated time, and when he is present, his presence is such that the *medical* reviews of Dickens's works mention him less frequently than do literary reviews.

Philip Collins's essay addresses basically the same characters as Leavis's, especially Eliot's Lydgate in *Middlemarch*, Kingsley's Tom Thurnall in *Two Years Ago* and Dickens's Allan Woodcourt and "Physician". Collins points out the reformist activity of which the "local practitioner was – or could and should be – at the centre." His supporting statements are, however, not always entirely accurate. For example, he says that Lydgate has "new ideas about . . . ventilation." The ideas actually were proposed by Thomas Sydenham in the seventeenth century and set into practice in the eighteenth.[12] Collins also says that "Fever is important in *Bleak House* . . . involving several characters." Fever *per se* is only mentioned in connection with the "fever houses" in Tom-all-Alone's; it does not strike any of the characters. Collins is of the opinion that the crossing-sweeper, Jo, dies of fever; I contend he was tubercular (or possibly asthmatic, see Chapter 5).

Collins cites Sir William Osler (1848-1919), who said that novels may provide more information than *The Lancet* on the "little everyday struggles and aspirations of the profession."[13] Dickens's novels do not stand out in this respect. We learn from Bob Sawyer in *Pickwick Papers* of the difficulties in establishing a practice, and the problems encountered by Woodcourt show us that things hadn't changed much over the intervening 15 years between the novels.

Dickens's medical personnel

Given the limited possibility of becoming a physician, noted above, it is small wonder that the majority of Dickens's medical men are surgeons. Consistent with common usage, his terminology is not always strictly correct, frequently referring to the man as "the doctor" after having identified him as "a surgeon."[14] There are some cases in which the proper classification is not clear, but only two figures - Parker Peps *(DS)* and "Physician" - are clearly identified as physicians.

Types versus individuals

Dickens created more than 2000 characters, of whom 50 or so are engaged in medicine in some way. While this is probably the largest single profession in Dickens's works, only Woodcourt and "Physician" are at all *professionally* important to the story. Most of Dickens's doctors - using the term for male medical personnel in general - can be classified by type: snobs, humbugs, money-grubbers or "good" doctors.

"Snobs"

The Anglo-Bengalee Insurance Company's medical officer in *Martin Chuzzlewit,* is an excellent example of the "practitioner as snob" type. John Jobling (F.R.C.S) shows off by holding an *ad hoc* lecture on anatomy:

> [I]n this portion of Mr Crimple's leg, there is a certain amount of animal oil ... If Mr Crimple neglects his meals, ... that oil wanes, and becomes exhausted. What is the consequence? Mr Crimple's bones sink down into their sockets, sir, and Mr Crimple becomes a weazen, puny, stunted, miserable man! (*MC*, 435/6)

and by throwing in a Latin phrase once in a while:

> *Bis dat qui citò dat* ("Classical scholar, Jobling!" thinks the patient, "well-read man!") (*MC*, 438).

None of this has any bearing at all on his competence – or lack thereof – as a medical man, but it is intended to impress the listener.

Another medical man in the "snob" category is Dr Parker Peps in *Dombey and Son*, whose practice - apart from the Dombey family - apparently consisted solely of titled patients, whose names he drops constantly.

"Humbugs"

The next "type" is what Q.D. Leavis termed the "self-important humbug."[15] One might expect a rather large number of such figures to issue from the pen of a satirist/caricaturist, and this expectation would be fulfilled, beginning with the early *Sketches by Boz*. The second chapter of "The Boarding House" introduces Mrs Bloss, a widow who

> having nothing to do, and nothing to wish for, . . . naturally imagined she must be very ill - an impression which was most assiduously promoted by her medical attendant, Dr Wosky . . . (*SB*, 292).

Dr Wosky was

> a little man with a red face - dressed of course in black, with a stiff white neckerchief. He had a very good practice, and plenty of money, which he had amassed by invariably humouring the worst fancies of all the females of all the families he had ever been introduced into (*SB*, 297).

He panders to Mrs Bloss:

> 'Our friend requires great care,' said Wosky. '. . .we positively must not give way to our sensibilities. We must take all we can get,' concluded the doctor, as he pocketed his fee, . . . and Dr Wosky rattled away to make fresh gulls of delicate females, and pocket fresh fees (*SB,* 297/8).

"Sir Tumley Snuffim" in *Nicholas Nickleby* is another humbug and more importantly, a flaunted status symbol. Sir Tumley never actually appears, we only hear of his great medical perspicacity from Mr Wititterly. Mrs Wititterly, like Mrs Bloss, indulges in "delicacy of health" and is even encouraged by her husband to do so. This undoubtedly strained Mr Wititterly's purse, but as Peterson points out: "It is . . . possible that the services of a medical man may have been one of the status symbols of the growing industrial and commercial middle classes in this period. . ."[16] And, of course, a knighted doctor as one's personal attendant was a status symbol of a higher magnitude. The aptness of Peterson's assumption is confirmed by the list of characters preceding the novel: Mr Wititterly is listed as "a middle-class gentleman."[17]

"Money-grubbers"

Disinterestedness was not a trait uniformly attributed by Dickens to doctors, and several "money-grubbers" appear (sometimes, like Dr Wosky, in the person of a humbug). The most prominent self-serving surgeon is the snob, John Jobling, of whom Dickens says:

> But Jobling was far too knowing to connect himself with the company in any closer ties than as a paid (and well-paid) functionary (*MC*, 437).

An incidence of anonymous "disinterestedness" is found in *Dombey and Son*. Mr Dombey, out riding, is thrown from his horse and injured. Taken to a public-house nearby,

> he was soon attended by divers surgeons, . . . who seemed to come by some mysterious instinct, as vultures are said to gather about a camel who dies in the desert. . . . One surgeon who lived hard by was strong for a compound fracture of the leg, which was the landlord's opinion also; but two surgeons who lived at a distance, . . . combated this opinion so disinterestedly, that it was decided at last that the patient . . . might be carefully taken home before night (*DS*, 635-6).

Both the landlord and the local surgeon stood to gain financially by Dombey's not being moved: the landlord by renting a room and providing food, and the surgeon by collecting fees, which he forfeits to Dombey's own medical advisors on his return home. Equating the surgeons with vultures emphasises the "disinterestedness" of the two surgeons who could draw no advantage from Dombey's accident.

"Good doctors"

The nameless surgeon who attends Lewsome at the inn in *Martin Chuzzlewit* is a representative of the anonymous "good" doctors: he "shook his head. It was all he could do, under the circumstances, and he did it well" (*MC*, 414).

A praiseworthy type of doctor is represented by Allan Woodcourt, the "good doctor" figure in *Bleak House*. Woodcourt is shown as a hero; not only in a shipwreck which is only reported, but more importantly for Dickens, I would argue, in his concern for the poor. As Peter Gay says:

> Allan Woodcourt is the doctor of every patient's dreams: always available, making house calls day and night, indifferent to money…[18]

One important "good doctor" figure is known only by his professional appellation – "Physician" in *Little Dorrit*. While others encountered in "society" at Merdle's dinners – "Bar", "Bishop", etc. - are snobs of the first water, Physician is said to tend poor and rich alike;

> Few ways of life were hidden from Physician, and he was oftener in its darkest places than even Bishop. There were brilliant ladies about London . . . who would have been shocked to find themselves so close to him if they could have known on what sights those thoughtful eyes of his had rested within an hour or two, and near to whose beds, and under what roofs, his composed figure had stood (*LD*, 683).

Here is a figure seen among snobs, but who is not one himself. Physician does not limit his practice to a wealthy part of town and to patients who can be expected, or are even able to pay. This portrayal has, as might be expected, given rise to considerable speculation about the "original" of the figure.

R.T. Young describes the various guests at Merdle's dinner and says that

> Dickens laughs at them all. But there is one of the company at whom he has no laugh, and that is the guest whom he names Physician, of whom he speaks in terms of such respect, admiration, and affection, that one cannot resist the impression that he must have had some particular person in his mind as he wrote.[19]

Young voices no speculation, however, as to who that "particular person" might have been. Dr J.E. Cosnett sees the figure as "almost certainly based on Dickens's friend, Dr John Elliotson, F.R.C.P.",[20] while Sir David Smithers assumes that the round table dinners given in the novel by Physician "were probably inspired by the Octave dinners given by the eminent surgeon Sir Henry Thompson, at which Dickens was at times one of the distinguished guests."[21]

Q.D. Leavis doesn't join in the "game" of identifying the original. Having discussed Trollope's Dr Thorne, and Eliot's Lydgate, she writes: "But 'Physician' in *Little Dorrit*, named generically like a character in a morality-play . . . is much loftier in conception than any of these actual physicians."[22] What she means by "these actual physicians" in referring to fictional characters is not clear.

Actors vs. supernumeraries

A review of Dickens's doctors yields a rather surprising picture. Most of the doctors he presents in any detail are not actually *professionally* important to the novel. A look at the prominent doctors and spontaneous associations with their names will illustrate this:

Dr Slammer *(PP)*	woos a widow; challenges his rival to a duel
Bob Sawyer (*PP*)	medical student, later debt-ridden practitioner
Losberne (*OT)*	family friend; retires from practice
Nameless (*OCS)*	humbug; prescribes what has been done
Jobling *(MC)*	abets fraud
Parker Peps (*DS)*	name-dropper
Chillip *(DC)*	meek, afraid of Aunt Betsey Trotwood
Allan Woodcourt (*BH*)	exception
Bayham Badger (*BH*)	brags about wife's first two husbands, representatives of the military might of the nation and scientific enquiry, respectively
Harold Skimpole *(BH)*	selfish and lazy; doesn't practice
Physician (*LD*)	exception
Dr Manette (*TTC)*	more important as a patient

The two "exceptions" here deserve closer attention. "Physician" was discussed above. In the case of Allan Woodcourt, we find that, with Bayham Badger and Harold Skimpole, he is one of a trio of doctors. The contrasts between the three allude to various aspects of Dickens's social and in this novel at least, socio-medical criticism. Dickens shows the three men differently with respect to their profession; one behaves as Dickens would expect from a worthy doctor (Woodcourt), one apparently does what is necessary, but no more (Badger) and one doesn't practice at all (Skimpole). The positive figure, Woodcourt, is the only one of the three mentioned outside Esther's narrative by the omniscient narrator, and also the only one who has reported dealings with patients. Although he assists in Badger's Chelsea practice, implying attendance on affluent patients (*BH,* 629), he charitably treats poor patients, like "Nemo" (Esther's unknown father, Captain Hawdon) (*BH,* 127). He also treats Miss Flite, a Chancery victim who lives in Krook's house (*BH,* 181), Jenny, the brickmaker's wife, whom he encounters by chance in London (*BH*, 577), and Jo, the crossing-sweeper (*BH,* 587). Lacking money and political connections, Woodcourt is unable to establish himself in practice in London. In what may be both a recollection of Smollett's Roderick Random[23] and a reflection of nineteenth-century reality, Woodcourt takes a job as a ship's surgeon. An intriguing passage is found in connection with Woodcourt after his return from India:

A brown sunburnt gentleman, who appears in some inaptitude for sleep to be wandering abroad rather than counting the hours on a restless pillow, strolls hitherward at this quiet time. Attracted by curiosity, he often pauses and looks about him, up and down the miserable by-ways. Nor is he merely curious, for in his bright dark eye there is compassionate interest; and as he looks here and there, he seems to understand such wretchedness, and to have studied it before (*BH,* 576).

This is, perhaps, a cameo role played by the author himself. Dickens frequently took long walks at night and not always in the best parts of London.[24] It may be that Dickens is here pointing to his perceived role as a doctor to the ills he saw in society.[25] The man is not immediately identified as Woodcourt, evinces both curiosity concerning his surroundings and compassionate interest which outweighs mere curiosity. This certainly applies as a description of Dickens, with his eager, inquiring mind, compassion for the downtrodden – and also his activities in the amelioration of wretchedness.

One of the novel's many coincidences brings Woodcourt together with Jenny and thus with Jo, and he learns that Jo had transmitted smallpox to Esther. For the first and only time, this model doctor displays repugnance in dealing with a suffering creature - whose repulsiveness has been emphasised through the whole novel and overlooked only by angelic natures like Esther and Charley, who pay dearly for their compassion, and by the lower orders like Jenny. But humanity wins out and Woodcourt sees to it that Jo is cared for. In such scenes, Dickens shows Woodcourt's importance to the message of the novel and his appropriateness as a partner for Esther in ameliorating the condition of England, even though his medical activity as described is not necessary to the plot. In the view of one doctor,

> The author pays a tribute to this physician as a man whom the poor loved; he endeavors to show him as charitable, kindly, brave, and indefatigable . . . but as a matter of fact, he is throughout but a lay figure used to develop and bring out the plot.[26]

This was apparently also the feeling of W.H. Maidlow of St. Bartholomew's Hospital, who writes that "the best of [his doctors], such as Woodcourt, Losberne, Manette, or Jeddler, might not have been doctors at all as regards their influence on the stories".[27] If disease and contagion were not so important to *Bleak House*, it would be possible to switch the young clergyman, Frank Milvey (*OMF*), and Woodcourt with very little imaginative effort, since Woodcourt's observed action is administering bread and wine and teaching Jo to say the Lord's Prayer. The defining characteristic of both men is selfless compassion.

Models in earlier literature

As the speculations about "Physician" above show, looking for the "originals" of Dickens's figures has long been a popular past-time – among both serious scholars and leisure readers. While certainly not a matter of weighty critical interest, I include some original thoughts here because it was long a considerable part of the medical reception of Dickens's works.

Apart from the broad hints he gives in *Martin Chuzzlewit* concerning Lewsome, Dickens identifies only one original among his medical personnel. But for seven of his more prominent characters and one secondary character, literary predecessors are plausible. The frequency with which Dickens makes reference to the works which he had read as a boy "sitting on [his] bed, reading as if for life"[28] is an indication of the importance of these works in the nurture of Dickens's imagination and creative genius. Identification of apparent literary models may thus be considered on a somewhat different level than the usual game-playing surrounding the purported "real life" models. It is possible here to discern underlying similarities in theme and the way in which Dickens incorporates his early reading into his own unique creations. Two each of these figures are taken from Shakespeare and Smollett, three from Fielding and one from LeSage.

Taking the "originals" in the order of authors listed above, the first of these Dickensian figures is Dr Slammer, surgeon of the 97th Regiment, whom the Pickwickians meet in Rochester. Of his capacity as a surgeon, Dickens says nothing. Dr Slammer is portrayed as being very sociable - he "took snuff with everybody, chatted with everybody, laughed, danced, played whist, did everything and was everywhere." (*PP*, 19-20) He courts a little old widow, whose "rich dress and profusion of ornament bespoke her a most desirable addition to a limited income." (*PP*, 20) The widow ignores him at the ball in the Bull in favour of Jingle, who was wearing Nathaniel Winkle's rather conspicuous Pickwick Club coat, resulting in Winkle's being inappropriately challenged to a duel.

> The stranger was young, and the widow was flattered. The doctor's attentions were unheeded by the widow; and the doctor's indignation was wholly lost upon his imperturbable rival. . . . The little Doctor thirsted for his life (*PP*, 20-21).

A literary model can be postulated for Dr Slammer, especially considering how often Dickens refers to Shakespeare. Dr Caius in "The Merry Wives of Windsor" hopes, at the start of the play, to improve his income by marrying a wealthy young woman, Anne Page. When Caius first appears (Act I, Scene 4), he learns that Sir Hugh Evans wants that young woman to marry Abraham Slender. Outraged by Sir Hugh's interference, Caius issues a challenge to a duel.
In support of the hypothesis that Caius was the model for Dr Slammer, it is noted that Dr Slammer's rival is Alfred Jingle, who is introduced as a thin man. Dickens makes this point again immediately before Jingle's encounter with the widow and Dr Slammer: Both the Pickwickian Tracy Tupman and Jingle would like to go to the ball which is beginning upstairs, but Jingle says his luggage "hasn't arrived yet" and he has nothing to wear. Tupman says: "I should be very happy to lend you a change of apparel . . . but you are rather slim, and I am -"

Jingle interrupts and says "Rather fat" (*PP*, 16). It seems implied that Jingle is (Abraham?) "Slender."

Several authors reviewing Dickens's doctors claim that Dr Slammer was modelled on Dr Matthew Lamert, who married Dickens's widowed aunt, Mary Barrow.[29] However, like many novelists, Dickens created new characters combining characteristics of people he knew or had observed. Indeed, he wrote: "I never represent an individual but always a combination of individuals in one."[30] Since Dr Lamert had a son James, and Dickens delighted in wordplay, it is not unlikely that [Jame] sLamer [t] stood godfather to the name and his father to the profession without any further similarities.[31]

Lewsome, a surgeon's assistant in *Martin Chuzzlewit,* is the other medical figure in Dickens with a predecessor in Shakespeare - and Dickens himself gives a clue to this. One of Jobling's snobbisms is citing "Romeo and Juliet":

> Your bosom's lord sits lightly on its throne, Mr Chuzzlewit, as what's-his-name says in the play.[32] I wish he said it in a play which did anything like common justice to our profession, by-the-bye. There is an apothecary in that drama, sir, which is a low thing; vulgar, sir, out of nature altogether (*MC*, 638/9).

In the original, Romeo hears of Juliet's "death" and decides to go to her tomb and commit suicide. Although he has been active with his sword for a good part of the preceding four acts, his choice falls on poison. He remembers seeing a poor apothecary and assumes, rightly, that the man can be bribed to sell him poison, although it is forbidden by law.

In Dickens's version, Jonas Chuzzlewit had gained power over Lewsome by means of gambling debts, which he agreed to cancel in return for Lewsome's procuring the "drugs", as he termed the poisons. He wanted "one that was instantaneous in its effect; of that he wanted very little and one that was slow, and not suspicious in appearance, of which he wanted more." Jonas pointed out that "He could get them without [Lewsome's] aid at half a hundred places, but not so easily . . . [which] was true" (*MC*, 738). In sixteenth-century Mantua, purchasing or selling poisons was already a capital offence. In Victorian England, traffic with poison was not regulated until the Pharmacy Act of 1868. The sale of certain poisons had been restricted earlier, for example by the Arsenic Act in 1851, but such Acts were objected to because the clauses and restrictions would interfere with trade of druggists and wouldn't stop murder anyway.

The death planned by Jonas Chuzzlewit is not occasioned by the poisons so obtained: Anthony Chuzzlewit, Jonas's father, dies a natural death of a stroke preceded by an epileptiform seizure (see Chapter 4). In the end, the similarity of the scenes is again noted: the character buying the poison commits suicide with it.

Tobias Smollett - a trained surgeon - was one of Dickens's early favourites, so it is no wonder that, in addition to the connections with Woodcourt, mentioned above, two of his medical figures appear to bear traces of Smollett's characters. The first is probably English literature's most famous medical student, Bob Sawyer in *The Pickwick Papers*.

Bob Sawyer and Ben Allen are first encountered at Dingley Dell, later in Lant Street (where the young Dickens lived while his father was imprisoned in the Marshalsea), and finally in Bristol, in a "newly-painted tenement . . . which a red lamp, projecting over the fan-light of the street-door, . . . announced as the residence of a medical practitioner. . ." (*PP*, 477). The practice had been offered for sale about the time Bob Sawyer qualified and his "friends came down with the needful". However, just having the practice didn't mean having patients, or specifically, paying patients. Advertising was not allowed, but stratagems were devised to call attention to the practice of "Sawyer late Nockemorf". While some critics scorn this behaviour, [33] "J.W.F". writes in the *Dickensian:* "If Bob's ingenuousness and the purity of his motives be . . . called in question, then let him be compared to Smollett's Captain [*sic*] Fathom, who made use of almost identical methods." But as J.W.F. points out, "Fathom was an unscrupulous villain, which is absolutely not true of Bob Sawyer."[34]

Peterson confirms Dickens's realistic description of a beginning practitioner.

> [He] had to have capital for the rental of a house and for the supply of drugs he would stock. He also needed funds to live on in the early years of practice. The first years were likely to be lean years. . . . Even when patients came in sufficient numbers, they did not usually pay cash.[35]

There was undoubtedly more outlay than income for many men in the early years after qualification, even though "[b]efore the twentieth century, there was no call for costly premises, expensive equipment and insurance policies."[36]

This is Bob's lament:

> It's wonderful how the poor people patronise me. . . . They knock me up at all hours of the night, take medicine to an extent which I should have conceived impossible, put on blisters and leeches with a perseverance worthy of a better cause, and make additions to their families in a manner which is quite awful. . . . [It's very gratifying], only not quite so much so as the confidence of patients, with a shilling or two to spare, would be (*PP*, 599).

Dickens also apparently "borrowed" Smollett's Roderick Random for the figure of Haggage in *Little Dorrit*. The reader is first introduced to the Dorrit family when Amy, or "Little Dorrit" is born. The doctor called in to attend the birth is an imprisoned debtor, who is drinking and playing cards when he is called:

The doctor was amazingly shabby . . . (he had been in his time the experienced surgeon carried by a passenger ship) . . . "Childbed?" said the doctor. "I'm the boy!" With that, the doctor took a comb from the chimney-piece and stuck his hair upright - which appeared to be his way of washing himself - produced a professional chest or case, of most abject appearance, settled his chin in the frowsy wrapper round his neck, and became a ghastly medical scarecrow (*LD*, 61).

Roderick Random was a naval ship's surgeon, not aboard a civilian passenger ship. Like Haggage, he had landed in the Marshalsea because of debt, where he became careless of his person - and that sounds familiar in the description above.

Another of Dickens's favourite authors was Henry Fielding. Dickens appears to have used three medical figures from *Tom Jones*. Writing in *The Dickensian,* T.W. Hill points out the similarity between the unnamed doctor in Fielding's novel and the one called in to tend Nell in *The Old Curiosity Shop*:

'I should give her,"said the doctor at length, 'a tea-spoonful every now and then, of hot brandy and water. . . . I should also,' observed the doctor, who had passed the footbath on the stairs, 'I should also,' said the doctor, in the voice of an oracle, 'put her feet in hot water, and wrap them up in flannel.' . . . With which parting injunction, slowly and portentously delivered, the doctor departed, leaving the whole house in admiration of that wisdom which tallied so closely with their own (*OCS,* 356).

Says Hill:

A delightful example of the soothing 'bedside-manner' of the general practitioner. After reading carefully this description, it will be amusing to recall the . . . passage from *Tom Jones*, Book VII, Chapter 13, with which Dickens was, of course, very well acquainted.[37]

One of the three doctors in *Bleak House* seems also to be based on a figure in *Tom Jones*. In Book I, Chapter 10 the reader learns that Squire Allworthy was hospitable, even to people in pecuniary difficulties:

Among others of this kind was Dr Blifil, a gentleman who had the misfortune of losing the advantage of great talents by the obstinacy of a father, who would breed him to a profession he disliked. In obedience to this obstinacy the doctor had in his youth been obliged to study physick or rather to say he studied it; for in reality books of this kind were almost the only ones with which he was unacquainted; and unfortunately for him, the doctor was master of almost every other science but that by which he was to get his bread; the consequence of which was, that the doctor at the age of forty had no bread to eat.[38]

He has a wife and children, but they are not with him during his extended stay with Squire Allworthy. They are, however, the reason he can't marry Bridgit Allworthy himself, but must call in his brother, Captain Blifil.

While it is well-known that Leigh Hunt was the overt model for Harold Skimpole of *Bleak House*,[39] the description of Dr Blifil brings Skimpole immediately to mind. Skimpole reportedly "had been educated for the medical profession, and had once lived in his professional capacity, in the house of a German prince" (*BH,* 63). He had "never been able to prescribe with the requisite accuracy of detail" (*BH,* 64), so he lost the job - which Skimpole frankly admits was justified - and had never practiced since. He has a wife and at least three daughters, whom he leaves to face the creditors while he dallies at Bleak House or anywhere else he can.

The secondary character for whom a literary model can be postulated is also taken from *Tom Jones*, and is as incidental in that novel as he becomes in *Little Dorrit*. Tom Jones rescues Sophie Western and breaks his arm in the process. The surgeon

> holding forth the broken arm, . . . began a long and very learned lecture of anatomy, in which simple and double fractures were most accurately considered[40]

While this reminds one of John Jobling's *ad hoc* lecture on Mr Crimple's leg, it also calls to mind the nameless surgeon at St. Bartholomew's Hospital, who treats the injured Cavelletto. In response to Clennam's question about the seriousness of the injury, the surgeon replies:

> 'Ye-es, it's enough. There's a compound fracture above the knee and a dislocation below. They are both of a beautiful kind.' He gave the patient a friendly clap on the shoulder again, as if he really felt that he was a very good fellow indeed, and worthy of all commendation for having broken his leg in a manner interesting to science (*LD*, 157).

The last of the figures with a postulated literary model is Dr Parker Peps in *Dombey and Son.* Peps is "one of the Court Physicians, and a man of immense reputation for assisting at the increase of great families" (*DS,* 4). A literary model for Peps might be found in Dr Sagrado, in LeSage's *Gil Blas*. Dr Sagrado "owed [his] reputation to resounding, empty phrases, his majestic presence and a few cases which had ended happily and had brought him more honour than he deserved."[41] In Chapter 47 of *Dombey and Son*, Dickens evokes a "good spirit who would take the house-tops off, with a more potent and benignant hand than the lame demon in the tale" (*DS*, 685). This refers to LeSage's tale *The Devil upon Two Sticks* (1707), which Dickens had read as a child, in a translation by Smollett, so the model assumption is plausible, since he apparently had LeSage in mind while writing *Dombey*.

Lest one think I am accusing Dickens of plagiarism, it should be noted that this sort of "borrowing" was apparently common. To cite just one example, Spottletoe of *Martin Chuzzlewit* can be found in Conrad's *Heart of Darkness*. The difference exists in the age at which the "model" was read and the facility with which not only a description, but situations and characters are woven into entirely new fabric.

Dickens and nurses

It would be impossible now to envision the medical profession without nurses. But nurses, in the modern sense, were practically unknown until fairly late in the Victorian period, although the situation began changing about 1840. One almost automatically thinks of Florence Nightingale (1820-1910) and her activities during the Crimean War in associating Victorian England and nursing, but there were at least two earlier institutions created to raise the standards of the profession in Britain. One was The Institution for Nursing Sisters, started in 1840 by the Fry Sisters, and the other St. John's House, founded in 1846. In these institutions, a "period of between one and three month's probationary training in a voluntary hospital was required before a nurse was admitted as a full member of the sister-hood; she was then guaranteed a salary, full board and free care during sickness."[42] Many women hired out as "monthly" nurses to tend women in childbed, but these were not generally trained professionals. As the medical historian Irvine Loudon points out, "Amongst the poor . . . the most common birth-attendants were the multitude of untrained and largely illiterate women who also did nursing, laying-out, and other jobs in steady demand."[43] Several such figures are encountered in Dickens's works. For the most part, however, nursing of the sick was a family matter and the sick-room the women's sphere of action. While this fact of Victorian life is not surprisingly brought out more strongly by the women novelists of the age, like Mrs Gaskell in *Cranford*, or Charlotte Brontë in *Shirley*, Dickens does make reference to it. In the *Sketches*, Dickens voices the common opinion:

> ... what hands, be they ever so gentle, can wipe the clammy brow, or smooth the restless bed, like those of mother, wife, or child? ("The Hospital Patient" *SB*, 211).[44]

A later example is found in *A Tale of Two Cities*, in Lucie Manette's account of the voyage home from France with her father:

> My father was so reduced, that I was afraid to take him out of the air, and I had made a bed for him on the deck near the cabin steps, and I sat on the deck by his side to take care of him (*TTC*, 101).

When there were no adept women in the family, nursing was sometimes the duty of a particularly trusted woman employee. For example, it is said of Mrs Rouncewell, the housekeeper of Chesney Wold, that

> If ever [Sir Leicester] were very ill, or if he were knocked down by accident, or run over, or placed in any situation expressive of a Dedlock at a disadvantage, he would say, if he could speak, 'Leave me, and send Mrs Rouncewell here!' feeling his dignity, at such a pass, safer with her than with anybody else (*BH*, 77).

And Mrs Rouncewell, fittingly at hand when Sir Leicester suffers a stroke, is entrusted with his care – instead of Sir Leicester's cousin, Volumnia.

There is one notable exception to the women-as-nurses trope. In *Great Expectations*, Herbert Pocket tends to Pip's burns and it is Joe Gargery who tends Pip in his illness after Magwitch's death. On the one hand, this is because there are no women close to Pip. On the other hand, the only nurture Pip has experienced in his life comes from these two men, so providing sickroom attendance is in keeping with their roles, despite male gender and lack of medical training.

Dickens does use "professional" nurses in one novel. The two most famous "medical" figures in *Martin Chuzzlewit* are nurses: Sairey Gamp and her erstwhile friend, Betsey Prig. Sairey is introduced after the death of Anthony Chuzzlewit:

> Mr Pecksniff had been to the undertaker, and was now upon his way to another officer in the train of mourning - a female functionary, a nurse, and watcher, and performer of nameless offices about the persons of the dead - whom he had recommended. Her name, as Mr Pecksniff gathered from a scrap of writing in his hand, was Gamp (*MC*, 310).

Sairey Gamp has a more distinct personality than anyone in the novel, with the possible exception of Pecksniff. Her language is extravagant and wholly unique, with neologisms sometimes requiring to be read aloud to be understood. In J.B. Priestley's view, such a drunken, incompetent nurse could have been described by any competent Victorian novelist, but "only Dickens could have given her the wonderfully daft dialogue".[45]

Mrs Gamp has a habit of praising herself and attesting to her own sobriety by quoting Mrs Harris - who is not only never seen, but who doesn't even exist outside Sairey's "references":

> 'Mrs Gamp,' she says, . . . if ever there was a sober creetur to be got at eighteenpence a day for working people, and three-and-six for gentlefolks - night watching . . . being a extra charge - you are that inwallable person' (*MC*, 316).

A possible "original" in this connection was mentioned in a notice entitled "Mrs Harris & Deputy" in *The Dickensian* of May 1971, p. 119:

> Mrs E.E. Duncan-Jones of Birmingham University has drawn our attention to an echo in *Martin Chuzzlewit* from an eighteenth century prose classic not usually thought to have influenced Dickens. She writes:
>
> The name of Mrs Gamp's unforgettable friend Mrs Harris is not a distinctive one. Still, it seems likely that her name and a little more may be traced to Dickens's remembering an incident in Richardson's *Pamela*. Here we find (Part II, Letter 1x) a Mrs Harris associated with midwifery, with an 'honest imposture' (Richardson's phrase) and with the device of building up a patient's confidence by employing an 'assistant' to utter 'great praises' of her principal. . . . The 'honest imposture' involves bringing into the house incognito a Mrs Harris, who is a midwife and 'a person of eminence in her own way.' (Dickens uses almost the same words of Mrs Gamp.).

Several pages of the novel are dedicated to the description of Sairey's mode of nursing, which consists in essence of making herself as comfortable as possible. Administration of medication *per os* is achieved "by the simple process of clutching [the patient's] windpipe to make him gasp, and immediately pouring it down his throat" (*MC*, 411).

Reading these passages about Sairey and remembering the Sketch quoted above, especially the phrase: ". . . hands, be they ever so gentle . . ." raises questions about hired nurses in the nineteenth century and about Dickens's intentions here. One clue is the aside about the "numerous" disciples of the "Prig school of nursing." Another clue may be found in old Martin Chuzzlewit's admonition to Sairey to drink less, be more humane, regard herself less and her patients more, and perhaps be a trifle more honest.

That Dickens was using the characters to draw attention to a prevalent and unacceptable situation is indicated in the Preface to the book version of the novel, dated June 25, 1844:

> [T]he commoner the folly . . . which an author endeavours to illustrate, the greater the risk he runs of being charged with exaggeration;

But although Mr Pecksniff will by no means concede to me, that Mr Pecksniff is natural; I am consoled by finding him keenly susceptible of the truthfulness of Mrs Gamp. And though Mrs Gamp considers her own portrait quite unlike, and altogether out of drawing; she recompenses me for the severity of her criticism on that failure, by awarding unbounded praise to the picture of Mrs Prig.

Confirmation of Dickens's portrayal is found in texts on the history of nursing, some of which are discussed below in connection with the reception of Dickens's works in the medical community.

Are there trends or development in Dickens's portrayal of medical personnel?

Critics have long divided Dickens's works into "early" (*Sketches* to *Chuzzlewit*), "middle" (*Dombey* and *Copperfield)* and "late" (*Bleak House* to *Edwin Drood*).[46] Philip Hobsbaum points out that "in the earlier novels of Dickens, plot coincides with Theme only by chance" while in the later novels "incidents, characters, strands of plot, lines of action, the pattern of symbolism and the evocative prose all subserve and act out the great Dickens theme: the individual against the System."[47] Hobsbaum - and he is not the only critic to do so - writes of the "darkening" of the Dickens world.[48] Although comic figures can still be found even in the least comic of the novels, the rollicking fun of the *Pickwick Papers* is not reproduced in the later works. The question of interest to this study is whether the medical episodes and personnel conform to this overall development. Does Dickens's attitude toward the medical profession appear to undergo any change, and if so, is the change unidirectional from light to dark?

The first doctors in Dickens's works are in the *Sketches by Boz,* which predate all but *Pickwick Papers, Oliver Twist* and *Nicholas Nickleby.* Some of the *Sketches* were written concurrently with these early novels, with the complete volume published in 1839.

In the *Sketches* themselves, our "null hypothesis" that the medical personnel parallel Dickens's works in general and go from "light" to "dark" would be rejected. The first series of the *Sketches*, headed "Our Parish" presents only one doctor in "The Four Sisters". Mr Dawson, "a surgeon, etc.", is called in to attend a birth, assisted by "a fat old woman" (*SB,* 19), the prototype of Sarah Gamp, who appears some nine years later in *Chuzzlewit.*

The second series of sketches, headed "Scenes" contains no medical personnel; the third series "Characters" brings the sketch entitled "The Hospital Patient" (1836). The patient is attended by a hospital surgeon and two "dressers" who "smelt strongly of tobacco smoke" (*SB,* 238) and may be viewed as the forerunners of the introduction to Ben Allen and Bob Sawyer at Dingley Dell (*PP*, Chapter 11).

The fourth group of sketches, headed "Tales" contains two stories with doctors. In the first, "The Boarding House" (1834), Dickens lampoons the "self-important humbug" type.[49] There is also a medical student living in the house, Septimus Hicks, a "poetical walker of the hospitals". These characters are not to be taken seriously. Two years later, however, Dickens wrote another sketch included in this section, entitled "The Black Veil" (1836). This introduces a nameless young surgeon who has set up practice, but has no patients. The tone of the sketch is serious: the surgeon's assistance is sought by the mother of a man who is to be hanged for an unspecified crime, since she hopes her son can be resuscitated.[50] It appears possible that Dickens got this rather macabre idea from Dr Buchan's *Domestic Medicine:* Part III, Chapter IX is "Of Suffocation and Strangling from Hanging, Drowning and other Causes," which gives instructions for thwarting suicide by hanging.[51]

The most famous doctors in the *Sketches* are found in a separate section entitled "The Mudfog and Other Sketches", published between January 1837 and February 1839. Here Dickens engages in anti-intellectualism and satirizes the British Association for the Advancement of Science, as he had done with the opening chapter of *The Pickwick Papers*. "The Mudfog Association for the Advancement of Everything" is divided into specialist sections. Section A is dedicated to Zoology and Botany and a discussion is reported concerning "industrious fleas", facetiously reflecting on the discussions current at the time concerning, among other things, infant schools for the labouring class, licensing of performers, and a system of retirement benefits (*SB*, 521-522).

Section B of the Association is devoted to Anatomy and Medicine. The "speaking" names of the doctors in this section, such as "Knight Bell," and "Dr Soemup", are a broad clue as to the seriousness (or lack thereof) with which Dickens was writing. The first doctor presented is Dr Kutankumagen (of Moscow), who reported on the cure of a man of "a virulent disorder" with "symptoms peculiarly alarming to any medical man" (*SB*, 524). The disorder was perfect health, of which the patient was admirably cured.

Also in this first meeting, homœopathy, introduced by Samuel Hahnemann (1755-1843) in 1796, is satirized and used to criticise the workhouse diet. The homœopathic principle is based on dilutions, called potencies, which can become such that no molecule of the original substance can be detected - even by modern methods.[52] The Mudfog Association hears of a publican rendered dead drunk with three drops of rum in a bucket of water.

A Member begged to be informed whether it would be possible to administer - say, the twentieth part of a grain of bread and cheese to all grown-up paupers, and the fortieth part to children, with the same satisfying effect as their present allowance.

Professor Muff was willing to stake his professional reputation on the perfect adequacy of such a quantity of food to the support of human life - in the workhouses; the addition of the fifteenth part of a grain of pudding twice a week would render it a high diet (*SB,* 526).

This sketch and the famous scene of Oliver Twist asking for more to eat were more topical than today's readers may realise. *The Lancet* of April 21, 1838 carried a scathing discussion of the "low dietary" in workhouses and the deleterious results for the inmates and thus society at large.[53]

After these tongue-in-cheek sketches, Dickens was less facetious in his writings in general. Speaking names are still found; in *The Pickwick Papers,* "Dr Slasher" performs surgery; mention was made above of "Dr Slammer", whose second at the duel was "Dr Payne". In *Nickleby* we encounter "Sir Tumley Snuffim" - but that is the last speaking name for doctors. Dickens's attitude toward doctors would appear rather benign. The self-serving and self-important doctors of whom he approves least are mostly in the early novels. *Dombey,* the first "middle" novel, does have the"self-important" Parker Peps, and Harold Skimpole appears even later in *Bleak House*, but he does not practice medicine. With "Physician" in *Little Dorrit,* Dickens apparently saved the best for last.

It appears clear that the development of medical figures in the novels, while not always unidirectional, does to some extent parallel the overall development of Dickens's art - starting with the comic figure of Dr Slammer and the seriocomic Bob Sawyer, and progressing via relatively harmless self-importance to the fraud-abetting Jobling, but ending with "Physician". The nurses go from the ideal "natural nurse" exemplified by the Marchioness in *The Old Curiosity Shop*, to Sairey Gamp, and return to Dickens's ideal in the late novels. It can be noted, however, that while the development reflects what might be termed a humour-to-serious trend, it does not reflect the overall humour-to-pessimism trend postulated by Goetsch and others. Dickens cannot be seen despairing of the future of medicine in his portrayal of its representatives or practices, as some critics would see him despairing of society in his portrayal of its institutions.

Reception of Dickens's works among the medical profession

An author's reception is an interesting facet of any secondary study. Especially when a profession is depicted by a layman, criticism might be expected to be particularly sharp. If a person trained in medicine - like Smollett or any other medically-trained novelist - writes about doctors or disease, one would expect the details to be accurate. The expectation might be misplaced when the writer is not medically trained. This is where Dickens stands out among lay novelists, which makes Dickens's reception in the medical world interesting. Reviewing the articles chronologically by publication date, the oldest article found was Dickens's obituary, published in the *British Medical Journal* of June 18, 1870. The writer began by lauding Dickens's accuracy, saying what a loss that a man with such talent for observation and so facile of description hadn't turned to clinical medicine. He went on to point out that Dickens's description of hectic fever had been quoted verbatim in two medical textbooks,[54] but ascribed the description of Nicholas Nickleby's dying cousin, Smike, to *Oliver Twist*.

On the same day, *The Lancet* carried a longer (and more accurate) obituary, highlighting Dickens's involvement in reforms, particularly that of the workhouse infirmaries in cooperation with and support of a *Lancet* Commission.

Initially, the articles in medical and hospital journals (and also in *Cornhill Magazine* and *The Dickensian*) deal exclusively with the personnel. In older publications, it is usually no longer possible to identify the writer. However, someone writing in a hospital journal is presumably professionally associated with that hospital, as are the readers who comment.

In some cases, a hospital bias is apparent. Dickens sometimes mentioned St. Bartholomew's Hospital, and the articles written by men at "Bart's" seem to be slightly more favourable than some of the others. But even at that, the writers are not all of one mind. The opinions range from "Dickens never really understood doctors" [55] to

> to a man of [Dickens's] intelligence and powers of observation, the hollow sham that lay beneath much of the professional veneer must have been only too patent, and he does not hesitate to lay it bare, but so delicately clothed the facts he exposed in a cloak of humour, that not even the most sensitive can take offence.[56]

Doctors

In *The Pickwick Papers*, most of the attention from the medical community centres on the two medical students, Bob Sawyer and Ben Allen. George Umber writes:

> Dickens must have been well acquainted with the general character of the class of medical students who at the period . . . walked, as it was termed, the London hospitals, for the portraits bear all the evidence of having been originally drawn from Nature.[57]

An article in *The Dickensian*[58] reports on a speech given at the London Hospital and Medical College, in which Lord Rosebery[59] said "that his generation had grown to manhood under the impression that all medical students were like Mr Bob Sawyer and Mr Benjamin Allen, dirty, drunken and unscrupulous." The writer in *The Dickensian* says this libels both Lord Rosebery's generation and the two students.

The article signed only "J.W.F.", cited above, appeared in *The Dickensian* in 1915. It begins by citing Lord Rosebery and asks how anyone could "hurl such awful epithets [dirty, drunken and unscrupulous] at these immortal and harmless comedians." The point is made that they were certainly no dirtier than the majority, since "before the advent of Listerism, corporal, domestic or communal cleanliness did not really exist." As for drunkenness, "[h]ad Bob Sawyer and Ben Allen been fanatically teetotal, or even sweetly temperate, they would have been quite out of place in *The Pickwick Papers* and besides, it was their only failing."[60]

It must be remembered that medical students were

> notorious as the wildest set in town, drunken, lecherous, making nights hideous with their pandemoniums. The bad name acquired by hospitals in the first half of the nineteenth century can be largely attributed to the reputation of their medical students.[61]

There was no student housing as such. "Collegiate residences" were first introduced in the early Victorian period by "medical faculties concerned about the students' unruliness and lack of discipline." [62] *Punch* described "steeplechases in the dissecting room, cheating on the Latin examination, flirting with the barmaid, gin-and-water until three o'clock in the morning" as the "stereotypical activities of the medical student of the 1840's." [63]

T.B. Layton, in an article entitled "Dickens's Medical Students" comes to an interesting conclusion concerning the hospital affiliation of Sawyer and Allen:

> Now it is clear from this [discussion of dissection] that Mssrs Sawyer and Allen were not at the same hospital, but they were in a position to work together on occasion. The only two hospitals at which such an arrangement has ever been possible are St. Thomas's and Guy's. . . . Surgery and Anatomy had been taught at St. Thomas's and Medicine at Guy's. This union had ended in 1825, but the students of each hospital were allowed to attend the practice of the other hospital until 1836, the year in which the *Pickwick Papers* began to appear.[64]

Interesting here is that the medical men writing these articles are thoroughly versed in Dickens's texts. While they largely ignore medicine *per se* in the articles, they do give considerable insight into details which might have escaped a lay reader's ken – like the cooperation between the hospitals, of which Dickens apparently knew.[65]

In 1970, the centennial year of Dickens's death, the Wellcome Institute of the History of Medicine sponsored an exhibition entitled: "Dickens and Medicine". The exhibition displayed books, manuscripts and paintings dealing with medical people known to Dickens, the public health issues in which he was involved, and topics referred to in his works. The introduction to the catalogue, written by the Institute Librarian, E. Gaskell, has a paragraph on "The Medical Student" which reads in part:

> One does not look . . . in Dickens's novels for a rose-coloured picture of the Victorian medical world; no more than one expects him to represent other professional groups, say lawyers, as being motivated entirely (or even largely) by disinterested impulses. This being said, even the most sensitive of doctors reading his novels today can still be grateful for the delightful portraits of the medical students Bob Sawyer and Jack Hopkins[66]

The authenticity of the characters is doubted in an unsigned article in the *Medical Journal of Australia* dated June 20, 1970. The author refers back to an article by Dr S. Squire Spriggs[67] which states categorically that

> Bob Sawyer and Ben Allen . . . are not portraits of students, and certainly not of medical students. The observations from life made by Dickens in his youth . . . were made in a humble stratum of society, where one young man in training for his calling was much like another.

But in 1979 Sir David W. Smithers was of the opinion that "Bob Sawyer [et al.] are so up-to-date in their talk, clothes and manners that they could (almost) be at Guy's or Bart's today." [68]

Considerable space has been allotted to these figures as a reflection of the situation in the articles. Several of the articles on doctors in Dickens made more mention of these two characters than of others - which is not surprising since they are probably the best known of Dickens's medical personnel.

Some articles showed particular interest in other specific characters. The nameless doctor in *The Old Curiosity Shop* who treats Little Nell was, for example, the object of some consideration in an article by R.T. Young in *Cornhill Magazine.*[69] He writes:

We have Dickens on doctors, in a quieter mood [than with Bob Sawyer], but all the same making merry at their expense, in a brief interlude interpolated into the last sad stages of the story of Little Nell. The shadow of death is already darkening over the tale. The one inevitable end is fast approaching, and it is as if Dickens (who lived intensely in his characters) was shrinking from the task which he knew to be before him. So, to give momentary relief to himself and his readers, he seizes on the collapse of poor travel-stained way-worn Nell by the roadside, to introduce the scene in the inn and the humorous description of the doctor who apparently didn't know much and still more apparently couldn't do much, but was sly and clever enough to throw dust in the eyes of the landlady and the little cluster of sympathisers, and finally to leave the inn with a greatly enhanced reputation for deep professional sagacity.[70]

Whether this accurately explains this scene is difficult to say. Certainly comic relief was not unknown as a literary device and was used frequently even by Shakespeare. But the scene occurs more or less half way through the novel and in his *Life of Dickens,* John Forster claims to have been "responsible for [the] tragic ending [of *The Old Curiosity Shop*]" by suggesting "about half-way through" that Nell ought to die to "preserve the purity of the figure".[71] Perhaps Dickens originally intended for Nell to be very ill and, in the way of Rose Maylie *(OT)* and Madeline Bray *(NN)*, recover to live peacefully with her grandfather and the schoolmaster. The introduction of the comical doctor might have been intended to foreshadow the fortuitous outcome. Unfortunately, few and only undated "Working Notes"[72] exist for this novel, so apart from Forster's statement, what Dickens originally intended with Nell remains unknown. In a speech given in Edinburgh on June 25, 1841, he said of the death of Little Nell:

> When I first conceived the idea of conducting that simple story to its termination, I determined rigidly to adhere to it, and never forsake the end I had in view.[73]

This does not necessarily contradict Forster's claim, nor is it by any means clear that the "termination" of the story was decided on at the outset of writing.[74] If Young's opinion is accepted, it would appear that with this doctor Dickens just couldn't resist poking a little more fun at the medical profession, even when beginning to terminate the existence of a popular character.

Allan Woodcourt in *Bleak House* receives sporadic and rather inconsistent mention in review articles. Although Woodcourt is the "hero" – in the sense that he marries the heroine at the end - he is not always viewed favourably. Many writers, like those quoted above, have found him too lightly sketched to be of any real interest. R.T. Young calls him "an admirable young physician"[75] and goes on to say:

[I]n Woodcourt we see Dickens *in earnest* about a doctor, in earnest and striving (not unsuccessfully) to bring into strong relief the skill, devotion, unselfish kindness, and heroism of a young surgeon.[76]

This reflects what Dickens himself wrote in a letter dated May 20, 1853 to W.J. Clement, a Shrewsbury surgeon:

I hope you will find Woodcourt's part in the end of the story in keeping with what pleased you so much. I think it will be pretty, and not ungraceful towards his profession.[77]

The latest comment I have found was in a recent book review by Terry Eagleton in *The Lancet*:

There are few impressive portraits of doctors in the 19th century English novel – Allan Woodcourt in Dickens's *Bleak House*, Tertius Lydgate in George Eliot's *Middlemarch* – but Woodcourt is as tedious as he is virtuous, and Lydgate is brought low by his eye for a pretty face.[78]

The articles cited illustrate clearly the subjective nature of interpretation and the fascinating diversity of opinion, which can perhaps be accounted for in considering the evidence on which the interpretations are based. They also underline the relevance of a medical reading of Dickens's works, which brings to light aspects perhaps not apparent to lay readers. It remains, however, that Dickens's medical practitioners are human, unglorified and with all the foibles and follies of humankind.

Nurses

As specific characters, the nurses also receive some comment from the medical profession. "H.L.S." at St. Bartholomew's Hospital writes, incorrectly, that Sairey was trained at Guy's. Sairey mentions Guy's as the hospital in which her husband died, but that would appear to be the only connection. Betsey Prig, on the other hand, is mentioned in the text as having been recommended by St. Bartholomew's to nurse Lewsome. One can only hope that "H.L.S." was being facetious in writing:

[H]ere again it is obvious that Dickens was doing his best to pay us a compliment. . . . Later on he talks of the 'Prig School' of nursing. Indeed, in some respects he displays remarkable insight. He knew that this Hospital had devoted attention to surgery - Mr Slasher makes a bow. He knew the honourable reputation of our nurses. Mrs Prig heads a school.[79]

T.H.G. Shore writes that "the character of his nurses are no doubt somewhat overpainted, but [Dickens] probably intended to throw some light upon what was one of the disgraces of the period." [80]

Unlike other purported "originals", something is known about the original of Sairey Gamp. In the Preface to the "Cheap Edition"[81] Dickens writes:

> Mrs Sarah Gamp was, four-and-twenty years ago, a fair representation of the hired attendant on the poor in sickness. The Hospitals of London were, in many respects, noble Institutions; in others, very defective. I think it not the least among the instances of their mismanagement, that Mrs Betsey Prig was a fair specimen of a Hospital Nurse; [82]

Forster adds the following information:

> [B]ut he might have added that the rich were no better off, for Mrs Gamp's original was in reality a person hired by a most distinguished friend of his own, a lady, to take charge of an invalid very dear to her.[83]

The friend referred to is the philanthropist, Angela Burdett-Coutts (1814-1906),[84] to whom *Martin Chuzzlewit* was dedicated. In a letter to her dated September 16, 1843, Dickens writes: "Pray tell Miss Meredith, with my best regards, that I have written the second chapter in the next number [of *MC*] with an eye to her experiences. It is especially addressed to them, indeed." [85]

Books and articles on the nursing profession have also mentioned Sairey Gamp and Betsey Prig, and while the figures are deplored, the justice of the representation is usually conceded. Sarah A. Tooley, for example, writes:

> Sairey Gamp and Betsey Prig, the immortal examples of the private and hospital nurse . . . have played an incalculable part in revealing the low status of nursing in the good old times, and to their creator belongs an honoured place in the roll of early nursing reformers.[86]

Tooley points out the prevalence of the untrained hireling nurse and reports that Sairey's taking Lewsome's pillow did not stem from Dickens's imagination, but reflected frequent behaviour of even hospital nurses. Sairey and Betsey were, Tooley concludes, not introduced for comicality alone:

> [P]eople who shook with laughter over the sayings and doings of Sairey and Betsey were unconsciously having their eyes opened to the abuses exposed.

There appears to be only one positive opinion on record: Sir Edward Bligh's "A defence of Mrs Gamp". Sir Edward claims that Dickens never alleges negligence on the part of Mrs Gamp in nursing either Lewsome or Chuffey. It was, he further points out (though not entirely accurately), Betsey Prig's methods which were rough and unkind. And as the final defence, he writes:

Voluminous indeed are the descriptions of the qualifications of a good nurse, but there is one simple final test. Those who study the clinical material of the Lewsome case will admit that, as the doctor said at the time, it was one in which nursing and nursing alone mattered. In that case, Sarah Gamp passed the supreme test of efficiency and skill - *her patient recovered.*[87]

Considering the description of Sairey's mode of administering medication, quoted above, and that her activities in caring for Lewsome consisted primarily in making herself comfortable, eating well and telling Lewsome to be quiet, it would appear more likely that her patient recovered *in spite of* Sairey, rather than as a testimonial to her "efficiency and skill."

Leslie Fiedler writes that Sairey "clearly reflects . . . Dickens's attitude toward nurses, both amateur, which she is in fact and 'professional' which she outrageously claims to be." Fiedler goes on to surmise that Dickens had

actually cleaned up Sairey a little, presumably to avoid shocking his genteel audience; portraying her ... as a celibate though alcoholic widow rather than a prostitute and/or bawd, as indeed many such Victorian nurses were.[88]

We have no basis for believing that the original mentioned by Forster was possessed of the characteristics purported by Fiedler.

Conclusion

Dickens's medical personnel have been discussed over a long period in a wide variety of literary and medical publications. Plausible literary models can be identified for several of these characters, underlining the importance of Dickens's early reading for his creative genius and imagination. The reception of these characters varies, but there appears to be no particular outside influence tending to inform opinion at any given period or impose any sort of uniformity on interpretation. Even those figures one might contend Dickens meant to be odious are not always viewed that way by readers, and we find acceptance – or even approval – of characters like John Jobling and Harold Skimpole. Considering the reaction of medically-trained readers to the characters can help to understand the degree of accuracy with which Dickens portrayed medical men and, of course, hired nurses. As Dickens himself pointed out in the Preface to *Chuzzlewit*, the reaction is subjective and the description will be accepted or rejected on that basis. While, fortunately, the Sairey Gamp species of nurse is rarely encountered in modern hospitals, it requires no great effort to find parallels to Dickens's doctors. The distribution appears to have remained constant with a small minority engaging in insurance fraud,[89] some pandering to the wealthy and the vast anonymous majority performing often thankless duties.

The situation is somewhat different with respect to the diseases which Dickens described very realistically. The fact to be kept in mind is that Dickens, with very little formal schooling at all, succeeded in describing medical detail to an extent rarely surpassed even by people trained in medicine. This is often overlooked by medically-trained readers and perhaps not even registered by laymen unfamiliar with the diseases Dickens was apparently describing. The objective in the next chapter is to provide a reference guide to the medical episodes in Dickens's fiction, including some medical information to assist the lay reader.

---

[1] Umber, (1912).
[2] Collins (1989), 119.
[3] Peterson (1978), 6.
[4] Peterson (1978), 9.
[5] Cartwright (1977), 46.
[6] Peterson, 11. This practice still holds today except that one would not expect an apothecary to make a house-call, as was apparently common in Victorian England.
[7] Rosenberg (1999), 163.
[8] For a detailed discussion, see for example Bynum (1994).
[9] F.R. and Q.D. Leavis (1970), 242-247.
[10] Collins (1989), 117.
[11] Leavis (1994 reprint), 243.
[12] Shryock (1948), 21.
[13] Collins (1989), 119.
[14] George Eliot was also inconsistent - in *Middlemarch,* Lydgate was a surgeon by training, but he is referred to as "the doctor". Thackeray was pointedly even less accurate in *Vanity Fair*: Becky Sharp reports of a marriage offer she had received from Mr Glauber, whom she calls "a young doctor," "a country surgeon" and "a country apothecary" all in one paragraph (*VF*,118).
[15] Leavis (1970), 242.
[16] Peterson (1978), 28.
[17] Neither Sir Tumley nor Mr Lumbey, who delivers the Kenwigs's sixth child, is included in the list.
[18] Gay (2002), 65.
[19] Young: (1934), 709.
[20] Cosnett: (*BMJ* 1992), 1542.
[21] Smithers (1979), 72.
[22] Leavis (1970), 247.
[23] Dickens definitely evokes Smollett's *Humphrey Clinker* in connection with Woodcourt's mother and her lineage: Tabitha Bramble tells her brother that he "was called after great-uncle Matthew ap Madoc ap Meredith, ... a gentleman ... descended in a strait line ... from Llewellyn, Prince of Wales." Everyman Edition, 195-6.
[24] See for example "Night Walks" in *The Uncommercial Traveller*, 127.
[25] Kaplan,(1988), 173.
[26] DaCosta (1905), 12.
[27] Maidlow (1917), 52.

[28] Forster (1899) I, 10.
[29] See for example Darwin (1952).
[30] Cited in Gamble (1998), 10.
[31] One reason for creating the name as postulated - if Dickens did so – might be that it was James Lamert who ran the blacking warehouse and gave the young Dickens the job he so hated, effectively putting him "in prison" while his father was in the Marshalsea for debt. Unfortunately for this hypothesis, the slang term "slammer" for jail is American and not coined until about 1940, according to *Webster.*
[32] Romeo, Act V, Scene 1.
[33] See, for example, Young, Note 19 above.
[34] "Bob Sawyer and Ben Allen vindicated by a doctor", *The Dickensian* 1915-16, 188-190.
[35] Peterson (1978), 91.
[36] Porter (1997), 348.
[37] Hill (1953) 137-142.
[38] Fielding, H (1749). 1985, 75.
[39] See for example Forster, II, 123/4.
[40] Fielding, H (1749). 1985, 195.
[41] Alain-René LeSage: *Geschichte des Gil Blas von Santillana* (1730). Translated 1981 by G. Fink, Version 1877, 126 (my translation to English).
[42] Summers In: Barry and Jones (1991), 137.
[43] Loudon (1992), 120.
[44] Compare this to Thackeray's "Ladies, what man's love is there that would stand a year's nursing of the object of his affection?" *VF* 512.
[45] Priestley, "The Great Inimitable". In: Tomlin (1969), 14-31; here 25.
[46] see for example Goetsch: (1986).
[47] Hobsbaum , (1988) 13/14.
[48] for example Goetsch, (1986), 144.
[49] See "Dr Wosky" above.
[50] Curiously such a case was reported nearly 40 years later in the *British Medical Journal* of February 26, 1870.
[51] Buchan (1828), 393.
[52] A letter from Dickens to Dr Frederick Hervey Foster Quin, the first homeopathic physician in England, written in French and dated May 26, 1847, was written on a small piece of paper, and Dickens apologized for its "homeopathic size!"(*Letters,* 5, 75).
[53] *The Lancet*, 1838: 56.
[54] Miller, *Principles of Surgery*, 2nd ed. (1850), 46 and Aitken, *Practice of Medicine*, 3rd edition (1866), 111.
[55] Article signed "H.L.S" in *St. Bartholomew's Hospital Journal*, January 1917, 43.
[56] Shore (1922), 109-112.
[57] Umber (1912).
[58] Vol. 8, No. 8, August 1912, unsigned.
[59] Archibald Philip Primrose, 8th Earl of Rosebery, 1847-1929; Prime Minister 1894-95.
[60] "J.W.F.", 189. [c.f. Footnote 35].
[61] Cartwright, (1977) 53.
[62] Peterson(1978), 81.
[63] *Punch*, I (1841), 184 in: Peterson, 40.
[64] *Guy's Hospital Gazette* 50, 1936:553-562.
[65] A similar observation is made in connection with "Pickwick Syndrome", below.
[66] "Dickens and Medicine", The Wellcome Institute, 1970, 4.
[67] *Australian Medical Gazette* 1, 1914:13. Spriggs was Wakley's biographer.

[68] Smithers (1979), 30.

[69] *Cornhill* was similar in design to Dickens's *HW* and *AYR*. Founded in 1860 by George Smith, Thackeray was the first editor. It specialised in serialization of novels, including those of Trollope, Collins, Gaskell and Hardy. It ceased publication in 1975. I have been unable to identify R.T. Young.

[70] Young, 710-11.

[71] Forster (1899) I, 140. My emphasis

[72] Elizabeth M. Brennan, in her Introduction to the Clarendon edition of *OCS*.

[73] Fielding (1988), *Speeches* 10.

[74] Joan Winslow, writing in *The Old Curiosity Shop*. "The Meaning of Nell's Fate" (*The Dickensian* 88, 1981:162-7) comments on the ending saying: "The more subtle techniques ... suggest through imagery that Nell has triumphed over Quilp and that her death is a happy entry into heaven ..." In this respect, one might, although Winslow doesn't, postulate Clarissa Harlowe as a model for Nell, with Quilp a dwarfish Lovelace. A connection between Richardson and Dickens is seldom discussed, but six years after publication of *OCS*, Dickens described the performance of the French actress, Rose Cheri, as Clarissa Harlowe as "a most charming, intelligent, modest, affecting piece of acting" (Jan. 24, 1847).

[75] though he is a surgeon.

[76] Young (1934), 709; original italics.

[77] *Letters*, 7, 86.

[78] Eagleton (2002).

[79] " H.L.S.", 44-5.

[80] Shore (1922), 112.

[81] This edition, commenced in 1847, consisted literally of cheap reprints of all the novels published to that point to provide affordable copies of novels.

[82] Reprinted in the Penguin Edition, 42.

[83] Forster (1899) I, 318.

[84] See Chapter 7, "Public Health" below.

[85] *Letters* 3, 562.

[86] Tooley (1906), 45.

[87] *The Dickensian,* December 1951, 40-42, here 42. Original italics.

[88] Fiedler (1985), 83-84.

[89] This is a recurrent problem in the German national health system, and reports of irregularities in billing under the British NHS have also recently been reported.

CHAPTER 2: The "Pickwick Syndrome" and other diseases

There are several identifiable physical disease entities and syndromes to be found in Dickens's fiction. One aspect of Dickens's writing which sets him apart from other novelists is his description of such diseases. Where others of Dickens's contemporary novelists make use of vague "illnesses" to serve the plot, Dickens's descriptions are founded in reality, as also seen by doctors. Four morbid states play a major role in the novel and are therefore discussed in separate chapters of this dissertation. Others, while described by Dickens in equally precise detail, are often found in a secondary character and not central to the story. Dr John Cosnett notes the description of "bizarre and abstruse syndromes" in minor characters, which he feels were "introduced in order to demonstrate their recognition."[1] Apparently Dickens could not resist drawing on his vast powers of observations and description, creating characters presenting with signs and symptoms which range (for the unaffected viewer) from the ludicrous to the grotesque, from discomfort to serious danger to health. Dr Robert Bethel expresses the common opinion that the descriptions resulted from Dickens's own observations. Bethel writes:

> [Dickens's] famous descriptions of now known clinical disorders, which found their way into many medical texts of the time, resulted from his studies of symptoms in others and in himself.[2]

The statement can be questioned: "studies" implies a more systematic investigation than Dickens appears to have made. His own symptoms – as described in his correspondence, for example – are also conspicuously absent from the novels (with the tentative exception of old Martin Chuzzlewit's illness). Nonetheless, the range of descriptions is extensive. Some of the morbid states occur in only one novel, a few find their way into two or more works. This chapter presents debilities, diseases and syndromes which are not essential to the plots. Kept brief and limited mainly to physical medicine, the complaints are described in Dickens's words. Reference is made to articles published in Dickens-contemporary and present-day medical journals and some medical information is given where appropriate. As an aid for the non-medical reader, Appendix 2 presents a glossary of medical terms.

Arranging these descriptions creates something of a dilemma. Logically, one might expect the descriptions and the diseases or debilities to somehow parallel the development of Dickens's art. That would mean, on the one hand, that the least serious disease/debility would appear earliest and the most life-threatening last. On the other hand, Dickens's development as a man and as an author should mean that his descriptions of illness also become more sophisticated. Neither assumption is correct. I have therefore chosen to begin with the Pickwick Syndrome, since it is the one disease in physical medicine[3] with direct reference to Dickens in its nomenclature and it appears justified to give it "star billing" in the list. The decision to arrange the remaining topics simply in alphabetical order results in apparent disarray, with the significant and insignificant in haphazard sequence and an unavoidable see-sawing between early and later works. But arranging the diseases by "organ system," or grouping them by serious/non-serious or by causality, which are the current state-of-the-art medical modes of classification, would be presentist and equally jumbled. Related states are not necessarily found in similar characters or under similar circumstances. Diseases used in more than one novel are found several novels apart, and it is by no means true that the first description of the state is more simplistic than any later one. The discussion of repeated diseases are arranged in chronological order of publication, which helps to illustrate this point. Integrated, symbolic use of morbid states does not appear to be a set feature of Dickens's works. Rather, he uses illness, injury or debility at will for melodramatic purposes, for political ends, to identify a character, even for humorous ends, and sometimes for no immediately apparent reason. What stands out is his realism, regardless of the situation in which he sets the description, regardless of its purpose or lack of specific, apparent purpose.

The "Pickwick Syndrome"

Dickens's first novel, *The Posthumous Papers of the Pickwick Club* (*PP*, 1836), or more commonly *The Pickwick Papers*, introduces an awe-inspiring array of characters, most of whom are not Pickwick Club members, but encountered by Mr Pickwick and his friends on their "scientific" peregrinations. Rare are those who can spontaneously name more than a few of these characters. The figure one would expect on nearly every list is Joe, the Fat Boy. Joe is introduced in Chapter 4 of the novel: "…on the box [of an open barouche] sat a fat and red-faced boy, in a state of somnolency" (*PP*, 46). He is a servant in the household of Mr Wardle, and possibly the most frequent phrase uttered by that gentleman is: "Damn that boy, he's gone to sleep again!" When Mr Pickwick asks if Joe always sleeps so much, Wardle tells him "he's always asleep. Goes on errands fast asleep, and snores as he waits at table" (*PP*, 51).

The description of Joe's medical complaint is scattered through the novel, presented in part whenever the Pickwickians have any contact with Mr Wardle. Sam Weller calls Joe "young dropsy" with reference to his obesity, "young opium eater" with reference to his lethargy, and "young boa con-strictor" with reference to his voraciousness. He also sounds like a present-day health advocate in warning the boy to sleep a little less and exercise a little more.

The last appearance of the fat boy is at the beginning of Chapter 54 and is typical. Joe has been instructed to bring a message to the lawyer, Mr Perker, and not to leave off knocking, for fear he might fall asleep. Mr Perker's clerk opens the door:

> The object that presented itself to the eyes of the astonished clerk, was a boy – a wonderfully fat boy – habited as a serving lad, standing upright on the mat, with his eyes closed as if in sleep. [The clerk] had never seen such a fat boy, in or out of a travelling caravan; and this, coupled with the utter calmness and repose of his appearance, so very different from what was reasonably to have been expected of the inflicter of such knocks, smote him with wonder (*PP*, 675-6).

One of the earliest medical descriptions in Dickens, this is perhaps not even recognized as such by most of the lay community. For example, the first issue of *The Dickensian* reprinted an article from the *National Magazine and Monthly Critic* of December 1837. The writer refused even to admit that the description could be believed:

> The fat boy we admit to be a caricature, yet he gives variety to the work ... he is very laughable, and his peculiarities, however exaggerated, in many situations give great drollery to the scenes. But what we have more to notice regarding him, is that which has been entirely overlooked by the critics. On a former occasion . . . we pointed out a canon, which we think must be always applied to works of imagination, viz extravagance is *inconsistent imagination*; poetry is *consistent imagination*, i.e. *consistent within itself*. . . .[T]he creation of this character is not true to nature (and it is immediately seen not to be), but it is consistent with itself throughout.[4]

The writer was apparently unaware that Dickens's description was not, in fact, imagined. Cases of obese people who fell asleep at inappropriate times had been reported well before Dickens created Joe. Dr John Fothergill (1712-1780), a well-known British physician, had reported on two cases, one who "had perpetual drowsiness, and . . . such a degree of somnolency ... that he could scarcely keep awake whilst he described his situation."[5] And, as the medical historian Howard Markel reports, fourteen years before *Pickwick Papers* was written, William Wadd (1776-1829), Surgeon Extraordinary to King George IV of England, wrote that the pulse of fat people was found to be weaker than in others and attributed to this the lethargy and sleepiness of obese patients.[6] However, Dickens's was the most complete pre-instrumentation description of the condition and in deference to his keen powers of observation - clinical as well as social – it has become known as the Pickwick or Pickwickian Syndrome.

There is some controversy concerning who first proposed the term "Pickwickian Syndrome". In his 1985 article on "Dickens and the Art of Medicine," Howard Markel raises the claim for William Osler (1849-1919), who noted the classic description in Dickens. S.J. London reports that the syndrome was first described in 1936, but without somnolence, and that when, 20 years later,

Burwell et al. noted that somnolence is, indeed, part of the syndrome, they proposed the term "Pickwickian". London further reports that "[t]he term was quite obviously provocative but received only tentative acceptance, until a number of pediatricians discovered the syndrome in children."[7] L.S. Geisler also attributes the term to Burwell et al. in 1956,[8] while Peretz Lavie credits Burwell et al. with the first description of the syndrome in 1956 but says that the term "pickwickian" was coined by Osler in the eighth edition of his book *The Principles and Practice of Medicine.*[9] Markus Herrmann reports on Osler and on an article published by Bramwell in 1909 which included the term "Pickwick". He goes on to voice some surprise that "the fact that the 'fat boy in Pickwick' referred to a figure in a novel by Charles Dickens appears to have belonged to the general education of readers of medical textbooks at that time."[10]

There also remains some controversy as to what entity is actually meant by the "Pickwickian Syndrome." Writing in the journal *Sleep* in 1992, Dr John Cosnett cites hypersomnia, but goes on to say that the term has also been applied to the sleep apnea syndrome (a new disease "legitimized" by Joe's description[11]), and that alternative or additional diagnoses of Joe's condition must be considered:

> Given the obesity, somnolence, overeating and periodic behavioural aberrations, in a young boy, it seems possible that he portrays a diencephalic syndrome, or possibly the Kleine-Levin syndrome, rather than the cardiorespiratory syndrome of extreme obesity.[12]

Later, writing in *The Dickensian,* Dr Cosnett retrenches somewhat and reports that the"prevailing medical explanation of Joe's problem is that Dickens was describing a case of cardio-respiratory syndrome of extreme obesity." [13] Then, in a recent article in *The Dickensian*, Cosnett states that "a diagnosis of diencephalic syndrome is, perhaps, more appropriate."[14] Since, according to consultation with a neurologist, the main common feature of the two is apparently periodic breathing, I am inclined to disagree.

According to the 1990 edition of "*Klinische Syndrome*" by Leiber, the Pickwick Syndrome is now defined as an extreme form of obstructive sleep apnea in extreme adiposity with specific pathogenesis and various etiology.[15]

As with other characters in Dickens's works, living models have been postulated for Joe. Most such theories are without substantiation from Dickens himself. As K.J. Fielding has pointed out, "there is a large class of 'phoney' originals, [which] rest on nothing but someone's say-so, and which go *against* the evidence."[16] Among these is a claim that an actor, Richard Cockerill, was Joe's original:

When lecturing before the Manchester branch . . . on "Dickens and his Friends", I (E.J. Collins) exhibited a letter of Gustavus Vaughan Brooke's, which I held as a mortgage for money lent to Charles Peace, the burglar and murderer, who was executed in February 1879. I had met him very shortly after his shooting P.C. Cox. He came to my school in order to give an elocutionary and whistling entertainment. He produced a book of letters, mainly theatrical, addressed to Richard Cockerill. He told me . . . that he (Richard Cockerill) was the original of the fat boy in *Pickwick* . . . Of course, I don't suppose for a moment there is any truth in his assertion. It was part of his disguise assisted by (probably) stolen letters.[17]

Edwin Pugh made the claim in his book *The Charles Dickens Originals*[18] that Joe was based on James Budden, whose father ran the Red Lion Inn in Chatham. Pugh does not cite any source for the information, saying merely in the preface that he had talked with Henry Fielding Dickens, Georgina Hogarth and Katey Dickens Perugini in preparing the book. James Budden makes another appearance in Arthur Waugh's article "The Fat Boy" in *A Pickwick Portrait Gallery from the Pens of Divers Admirers of the Illustrious Members of the Pickwick Club, Their Friends and Enemies*, published in London in 1936. Waugh's source, however, was apparently Pugh. The unsubstantiated claim was used more recently by Dr M.H. Kryger in his article on sleep apnea.[19]

Assuming the existence of James Budden, we may permit ourselves the further assumption that he was obese - but this alone does not constitute the syndrome (or it would have a much greater prevalence than it does!) Dickens's description, which includes most if not all of the characteristics of this syndrome, precedes publication in medical journals by some 120 years. The curious part is that if indeed Budden was the original, the observations were made by Dickens at the tender age of about 8! Like so many other diseases realistically described by Dickens, it is not possible to know *where* or even *when* he made the observations.

Joe's only moment of importance, as far as the very loose "plot" of the novel is concerned, is the one time he is awake and spoils Tracy Tupman's wooing of Miss Rachael Wardle, which leads to her elopement with Jingle. Apart from this one episode, Dickens appears to have included Joe in the novel for the reasons postulated in the *Dickensian* article cited above: he is laughable and adds drollery to the scene. His disease served to identify him in the serial publication.

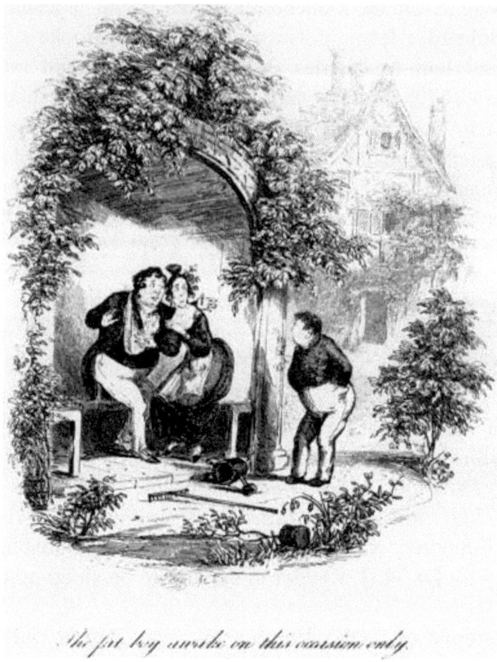

Fig. 3: "The fat boy awake on this occasion only." *Pickwick Papers*. The Dickens Museum.

Asthma

The term "asthma" is of ancient origin and was used even by Homer.[20] According to a nineteenth-century medical encyclopaedia, the term asthma "defines in general every form of laboured breathing, but more specifically, a definite disease in which there is temporary, usually periodically recurrent constrictive shortness of breath".[21] According to Dr Marshall Hall (1790-1857), in a lecture reported in *The Lancet* of April 21, 1838, "spasmodic" or bronchial asthma is a disease of the nervous system. It is to be differentiated from croup-like or laryngeal asthma, but "a morbid state of the stomach induces both."[22]

Asthma is first specified by Dickens in Mr Omer, the undertaker in Yarmouth (*DC*). Mr Omer is described as being "so fat that he was obliged to pant some time before he could say [anything]" (100). When David visits Yarmouth with Steerforth some years later, Omer's daughter Minnie tells David that "the weather don't suit his asthma out of doors" (247). In Chapter 30, when David returns to Yarmouth because Barkis is dying, he visits Mr Omer. Mr Omer asks if David minds that he smokes and when David says that pipe smoke is pleasant

– in someone else's pipe. Mr Omer replies: "What, not in your own? . . . All the better, sir. Bad habit for a young man. . . . I smoke, myself, for the asthma" (*DC*, 356).

Knowing the effect of smoking on the lungs makes this appear a rather strange treatment for asthma – or any disease entailing shortness of breath! But Dr Hall's lecture, cited above, makes the claim that "[a]s certain additions to the atmosphere induce asthma, so certain others, as the smoke of tobacco . . . relieve the disease." [23]

Consultation with a cardiologist confirmed my suspicion that Omer's "asthma" was probably to be understood in the first, general, sense of the nineteenth-century definition cited above. Omer would seem more to be suffering from an obstructive pulmonary or cardiac disease than asthma in today's narrower definition of "a disease of the airways that is characterized by increased responsiveness of the tracheobronchial tree to a multiplicity of stimuli"[24] (including nicotine). Nonetheless, when the paediatrician Dr Norman Jacoby was consulted to treat asthma in one of Dickens's descendents, he became intrigued with the possibility that Dickens himself may have suffered from asthma. In an article entitled "Charles Dickens' Asthma" [25] Jacoby writes:

> If [Dickens] suffered from asthma, why did he not write about it in his books? The answer to that is that he did and at great length – probably devoting more space to it than to any of the many other diseases he described.[26]

As Jacoby points out, there is no literary need for Mr Omer to have suffered any disease at all, and

> probably the condition was foisted onto him for no other reason than a wish to describe it. . . . In contrast to those highly accurate descriptions, [Dickens's] efforts with Mr Omer's asthma are poor . . . The answer is surely that he was describing a disease as he observed it in himself.[27]

What Dr Jacoby apparently overlooks is the uncertain nature of the term "asthma" at the time Dickens was writing. This may be simply a case of Jacoby's finding what he was looking for – a phenomenon we encounter several times in the interpretation of literature, not only by medical experts.

Jacoby also points out that David Copperfield, after chasing the young man who stole his box and his money ". . . sat down on a doorstep . . . with hardly breath enough to cry for the loss of my box and half-guinea" (*DC*, 145). Since *David Copperfield* is largely autobiographical, this would appear to Jacoby to support his claim that Dickens may have been asthmatic in today's sense of the term.

Another specifically "asthmatic" character is Mr Sleary, introduced in Chapter 6 of *Hard Times* as follows:

> Last of all appeared Mr Sleary: a stout man as already mentioned, with one fixed eye and one loose eye, a voice (if it can be called so) like the efforts of a broken old pair of bellows, . . ."Thquire!", said Mr Sleary, who was troubled with asthma, and whose breath came far too thick and heavy for the letter s,. . .(*HT*, 77).

Dr Jacoby says this is a "fair description of an asthmatic's wheezy breathing" and points out that according to the biographer, Peter Ackroyd, Dickens also lisped, though not as markedly as Sleary. Jacoby's conclusion is that

> It seems that Dickens was extremely vain in matters connected with his health, and if he went that far to suppress any knowledge of these conditions [gout, shortsightedness], surely he was doing the same thing for his asthma? On the other hand, it seems that he was not averse to transferring his own afflictions anonymously to his characters.[28]

While it would be difficult to deduce any particular similarity between Dickens and the undertaker, Mr Omer, there is reason to see Dickens in the figure of Mr Sleary. As R. Fowler pointed out:

> These difficulties ('th'-lisps) do not guarantee that what Sleary says is of any great interest; but the fact that Dickens has placed these difficulties in our way indicates that Slearly is *meant* to be listened to, that he is designed as a significant voice against Gradgrindism[29] in the polyphonic structure of the book.[30]

Indeed, Mr Sleary's function in society is to provide amusement for the people to offset their workaday world, in which the Gradgrinds and M'Choakumchilds do their best to stifle imagination and fantasy. Dickens, while providing social criticism, also wrote to entertain.

We find a possible hint of support for Jacoby's theory of Dickens's suffering from asthma in his correspondence. In a letter to J.P. Harley, written February 18, 1844, Dickens says: "To day I am neither useful nor ornamental – simply stupid, drowsy, sniveling, ugly, red-nosed, water-eyed, and gasping."[31] On March 20, 1844, Dickens wrote to Samuel Rogers: "I have a very red nose myself, and wheeze incessantly."[32]

Gasping and wheezing are not typical symptoms of a cold, and it is noted that Dickens does not specifically complain of a cold. Perhaps this is evidence for Jacoby's theory?

There is one character who says "I'm rather thick in the breath" who was not mentioned by Jacoby, though as with Sleary, a case could be made for some identification with Dickens. This is "The Golden Dustman," Noddy Boffin, in *Our Mutual Friend.* It may be postulated that Dickens saw himself as a sort of "Golden Dustman," taking the ugliness of the city and society and transforming it into a work of art. Despite the game of "find Dickens" which has resulted in his being identified in all sorts of characters, there has been no mention of this possible connection, but it appears plausible.

Ataxic Gait

In *Dombey and Son,* Edith Granger's cousin, Feenix, is described as being "not exactly certain when he walks across a room, of going quite straight to where he wants to go" (*DS,* 464). Cousin Feenix gives the bride away and "meaning to go in a straight line, but turning off sideways by reason of his wilful legs, gives the wrong woman to be married to this man, at first…" (*DS*, 468).

Apparently Cousin Feenix suffers from locomotor ataxia, or *tabes dorsalis*. This inability to coordinate voluntary muscular movements is the result of acquired syphilis and usually appears in patients in their 40s or 50s. Whether Dickens knew the origin is perhaps doubtful. Dr Alfred Fournier (1832 –1915) first affirmed the syphilitic origin of *tabes dorsalis* in 1875 in Paris, though it was at least suspected earlier.[33] Nonetheless, the debility is extremely fitting for the character: though a basically decent man, Feenix would likely have been a high-living Regency[34] dandy who lives abroad, having squandered his fortune as a young man. A debility arising from venereal disease would seem an appropriate comical and metaphorical identifier for a member of the effete aristocracy, which has lost its sense of direction in confronting the new plutocracy.

Blindness

Given the great potential for symbolism inherent in blindness, it surprises somewhat that Dickens made rather little use of it. There are only two blind characters, and the cause is not identified in either case. The first is Bertha Plummer, a poor toymaker's daughter in *The Cricket on the Hearth*, the Christmas Book for 1845. Bertha is physically blind and also kept "in the dark" about her father's poverty and ill-use by his employer.

The second blind character is Stagg in *Barnaby Rudge*. Barnaby's father, who was thought to have been killed with his master (but was himself the murderer) takes lodgings with Stagg and sends him to extort money from Barnaby's mother. By way of introducing his demands, Stagg says:

> There are various degrees and kinds of blindness, widow. There is the connubial blindness, ma'am, ... which is a kind of wilful and self-bandaging blindness. There is the blindness of party, ma'am, and public men, which is the blindness of a mad bull in the midst of a regiment of soldiers clothed in red. There is the blind confidence of youth, . . . and there is that physical blindness, ma'am, of which I am, contrairy to my own desire, a most illustrious example. Added to these, ma'am is that blindness of the intellect, of which we have a specimen in your interesting son, and which, having sometimes glimmerings and dawnings of the light, is scarcely to be trusted as a total darkness (*BR*, 422).

Dickens also lodges a protest against the perception of blind people by some sighted people:

> Why do you expect me, being in darkness, to be better than men who have their sight – why should you? . . . It's the cant of you folks to be horrified if a blind man robs, or lies, or steals; oh yes, it's far worse in him, who can barely live on the few halfpence that are thrown to him in streets, than in you, who . . . are not dependent on the mercies of the world. A curse on you! You who have five senses may be wicked at your pleasure; we who have four, and want the most important, are to live and be moral on our affliction. The true charity and justice of rich to poor, all the world over! (*BR*, 429)

The hangman, Dennis, turns traitor on the rioters at the end in an attempt to save his own life. Stagg, whose hearing is more acute as a result of his blindness, hears the soldiers' approach, tries to flee, but is shot.

Other ocular disorders

Dickens often describes the eyes of his characters. If the eyes are small, like Noah Claypole's in *Oliver Twist*, or close-set like Rigaud's in *Little Dorrit*, nothing good is to be expected of the character. This is a common melodramatic stereotype going back to Lavater[35] which Dickens, like other authors,[36] unhesitatingly used. "Lavater's view, as evident from a portrait analysis of his, [was] that small eyes bespeak a narrow-minded, uncouth person."[37]

One villain in *Nicholas Nickleby* is particularly recognized by his ocular characteristic:

> Mr Squeers's appearance was not prepossessing. He had but one eye, and the popular prejudice runs in favour of two.[38] The eye he had was unquestionably useful, but decidedly not ornamental" (*NN*, 30).

The eye might have been lost as the result of an accident, since the description continues: "The blank side of his face was very much wrinkled and puckered up." But his daughter, Fanny, has the same ocular characteristic.

A condition which is repeated in several characters is that of having one fixed and one normal eye. For example, Newman Noggs, Ralph Nickleby's clerk in *Nicholas Nickleby,* has "two goggle eyes, whereof one is a fixture" (*NN,* 8). Dickens does not seem to associate this condition with any particular character trait, since Noggs is a benevolent man (like Sleary [*HT*]; see "Asthma"), while the next such character is the dishonest real estate agent who sells young Martin Chuzzlewit land in Eden. Scadder's "grey eyes lurked deep within [his] head, but one of them had no sight in it, and stood stock still" (*MC*, 352).

One further character thus afflicted is Bunsby in *Dombey and Son*. In this marine-theme novel, Bunsby is described as having "one stationary eye . . . and one revolving one on the principle of some lighthouses" (*DS*, 353).

Clubfoot

In *The Old Curiosity Shop*, both Abel Garland and his son suffer from clubfoot, or *talipes*:

> Mr Abel, . . . looked nearly of the same age as his father, and bore a wonderful resemblance to him in face and figure . . . In . . . the neatness of the dress, and even in the club-foot, he and the old gentleman were precisely alike (*OCS*, 120).

This congenital deformity of the foot has been known since antiquity, but the pathogenesis is still unclear. Some forms are correctible, which was recognized by the Hippocratic school.[39] Whether the Garlands suffered a form unamenable to correction or why no correction had been made cannot be ascertained. It would appear that Dickens had somewhere seen such a father and son and was stuck by the curiosity. Since the deformity is congenital but not considered genetic, the chance of its appearance in successive generations is quite small.

Deafness

Like blindness, deafness is a debility, not a disease. It may be the result of disease, old age or trauma and Dickens makes use of all these possibilities, with old age the most prevalent. This debility is found in more than one character in some novels, but the cause of the debility, the form it takes and its role vary.

The first character encountered is Mr Wardle's mother at Dingley Dell (*PP*). She is described as a "very old lady" who uses an ear-trumpet. When Mr

Pickwick is introduced, she says more than once that she "can't hear him". Miss Isabella Wardle, the old lady's granddaughter, tells Pickwick "Grandma's rather put out now, but she'll talk to you presently." Later, there is some general conversation and Mrs Wardle asks what the conversation is about ". . . in a very audible voice; for, like many deaf people she never seemed to calculate on the possibility of other persons hearing what she said herself" (*PP,* 141). When a card game is proposed, Wardle says his mother's "very fond of a rubber" and asks his mother if that is not so. "The old lady, who was much less deaf on this subject than on any other, replied in the affirmative." So Dickens was aware of the "selective deafness" of old age which let the old woman hear only what she wanted to hear.

There is a second deaf character in the novel, an old man observed by Pickwick on the pauper side of the Fleet prison:

> On the opposite side of the room an old man was seated on a small wooden box . . . A young girl – his little grand-daughter – was … endeavouring . . . to engage his attention; but the old man neither saw nor heard her. … His limbs were shaking with disease, and the palsy had fastened on his mind (*PP,* 534).

Given the paucity of clinical information, "shaking with disease" could indicate Parkinson's disease, though it is by no means the only disease associated with tremors. The passage can also be interpreted to mean that the man is physically blind and deaf, which are not part of Parkinson's. Since, however, Dickens states that "the palsy had fastened on his mind," it would appear likely that his blindness and deafness were a consequence of dementia or severe depression, rather than physical in nature.

One extremely deaf old woman appears in *Nicholas Nickleby.* This is Peg Sliderskew, housekeeper to Arthur Gride. Gride complains: "She can never hear the most important word, and hears all the others!"(*NN*, 702-3) This might be taken as the "selective deafness" mentioned above, except that Peg is really so deaf that her responses to anything said at normal volume are frequently inappropriate. For example, when Squeers, acting for Ralph Nickleby, goes to her room to get possession of the papers Peg stole from Gride, he says that he has come according to his promise. Peg's response is: "So they used to say in that part of the country I come from; . . . but I think oil's better" (*NN*, 750). Dickens appears to be having some slightly malicious fun at the expense of an unpleasant old hag.

In 1979, Dr Ahmes L. Pahor discusses Dickens's use of noise deafness in his article "Charles Dickens and the Ear, Nose, and Throat"[40]. He contrasts the noise to which the Pickwickians were exposed in an open space during army exercises in Chatham (Chapter 4) with the noise in a closed room which permanently deafened Miss Pross in *A Tale of Two Cities* (Chapter 14). "Charles Dickens," writes Pahor, "would not realize the importance of his observations from a scientific medical standpoint, but the fact remains that he has described nothing that is not in keeping with present otological knowledge."[41] Undoubtedly medical science had, in the century between Dickens and Pahor, discovered the mechanisms involved, but it is astounding that there was nothing which needed correction in Dickens's descriptions.

In *Bleak House,* Dickens makes reference to the fact that hearing is the last sense to be lost by dying people. Jo, the crossing sweeper, is dying and tells Allan Woodcourt that "it's turned wery dark. . . . I hear you, sir, in the dark" (*BH,* 596). Pahor points out the correctness of the observation and that the sequence of loss is the same as in patients under anesthesia: "taste and smell are lost first, sight next, and hearing last."[42]

Great Expectations shows deafness first as a result of trauma. One of the debilities resulting from Orlick's attack on Mrs Joe was impaired hearing (*GE,* 98). More details of Mrs Joe's condition are given in the section on head injuries.

The second deaf character in the novel is Wemmick's father or "Aged Parent," who is described as "a very old man in a flannel coat: clean, cheerful, comfortable, and well cared for, but intensely deaf." Wemmick asks Pip to nod at the old man, as the only means of communication. The only thing the "Aged P." says he can hear is the small cannon which Wemmick sets off every evening at nine. The "Aged P." heats the poker, with which Wemmick fires the cannon:

> [Wemmick] took [the poker], and went out, and presently the Stinger went off with a Bang that shook the crazy little box of a cottage as if it must fall to pieces, . . . Upon this, the Aged – who I believe would have been blown out of his arm-chair but for holding on by the elbows – cried out exultingly.
>
> "He's fired! I heerd him!" and I nodded at the old gentleman until it is no figure of speech to declare that I absolutely could not see him (*GE*, 162).

Whether in fact the old gentleman heard the cannon, or whether perception was only the shockwaves that would have "blown him out of his arm-chair" is an unanswerable question. Dickens let the sensation – whatever it was – be the old man's greatest pleasure and portrayed a cheerful, uncomplaining soul in spite of a serious disability.

Going beyond the deafness of trauma or age, there are two deaf and dumb children, the first in *Bleak House*. Caddy Jellyby Turveydrop has a "poor little mite" of a daughter (Chapter 50), of whom Esther only reports at first that she is unresponsive when her father played music to amuse her.

> [Prince] would sometimes take the kit from his pocket and play a chord or two to astonish the baby – which I never knew it to do in the least degree, for my tiny namesake never noticed it at all (*BH*, 627).

It is implied in the text that Caddy had a difficult pregnancy, so the suspicion is raised that the little girl is somehow disabled. This is finally explained in Chapter 66, "The Close of Esther's Narrative", when Esther writes:

> I had almost forgotten Caddy's poor little girl. She is not such a mite now; but she is deaf and dumb. I believe there never was a better mother than Caddy, who learns, in her scanty intervals of leisure, innumerable deaf and dumb arts, to soften the affliction of her child (*BH*, 806).

The second deaf and dumb child is Sophy, the adopted daughter of the cheapjack Doctor Marigold, in the Christmas story for 1865. Marigold describes his first encounter with the girl:

> I come upon the poor girl who was deaf and dumb. At first look I might almost have judged that she had escaped from the Wild-Beast Show; but at the second I thought better of her, and thought that if she was more cared for, and more kindly used, she would be like my child (*Marigold*, 454).

Pahor speculates that Dickens may have had scarlet fever in mind as the cause of Sophy's deafness, which was either congenital, like little Esther's, or acquired very early in life. He cites the otologist J. Toynbee in saying that "scarlet fever was considered the most common cause of deafness and dumbness."[43] Marigold applies the same teaching methods which Dickens described in *American Notes*, Chapter 3 in connection with Dr Howe at the Perkins Institute for the Blind in Boston and his pupil, Laura Bridgman – who was deaf as a result of scarlet fever.

Dizziness

There is a secondary character in *Bleak House* with an unclear disorder. Phil Squod, assistant to Mr George at the shooting gallery,

> has a curious way of limping round the gallery with his shoulder against the wall, and tacking off to the objects he wants to lay hold of, instead of going straight to them . . . (*BH*, 279).

Phil's anamnesis, in his own words, includes

> Blowing the fire with my mouth when I was young, and spileing my complexion, and singeing my hair off and swallering the smoke; and . . . running against hot metal . . . a dozen years in a dark forge . . . and . . . being scorched in an accident at a gas-works; and . . . being blowed out of winder, case-filling at the fire-work business . . . (*BH*, 337).

Howard Markel postulates that Phil may have suffered Menière's disease, first described by Prosper Menière (1799-1862) in Paris some nine years after publication of *Bleak House*.

> The combination of Phil's intense dizzy spells and the loud noises he hears presents as a type of dysfunction of the vestibular nerve (cranial nerve VIII), most likely Ménière's [sic] disorder.[44]

This diagnosis can be contested, among other things on the basis of the textbook *Controversial Aspects of Ménière's Disease,* which states that this disease varies widely in severity and is characterized by vertiginous episodes.

> The symptoms may last for an hour or more, and then either subside completely or continue as a sensation of unsteadiness for some hours or days. Periods of longer than 24 hours of persistent spinning make the diagnosis of Ménière's disease doubtful.[45]

Since Phil must always lean against the wall for balance, it would appear that he did not suffer Menière's disease. Considering his history, traumatic damage to the inner ear would appear more likely. Phil is a good example of the meticulous detail with which Dickens described even secondary characters.

Dwarfism

Dwarfism, or achondroplasia, "the most common and best-known form of short-limbed, short stature"[46] is to be found in two of Dickens's novels. The first character is the villain of *The Old Curiosity Shop.* Daniel Quilp is described as an

> elderly man of remarkably hard features and forbidding aspect, and so low in stature as to be quite a dwarf, though his head and face were large enough for the body of a giant (*OCS*, 26/7).

Described by John Romano as a "rapacious dwarf, with his much apparent fairy-tale ancestry,"[47] Quilp's dwarfed, misshapen body serves as an outward sign of his misshapen mind. As Stainley Wainapel writes, "Dickens uses physical disability and deformity as effective metaphors for aspects of the human condition which excited his sympathies or indignation."[48] Quilp is portrayed as sexually attractive (perhaps the oft-cited attraction of repulsion?). His sexuality is made part of his ugliness and perversity, since he leers at Nell, offering to make her the second Mrs Quilp, should the first one die. As befits the fairy-tale ambience of *The Old Curiosity Shop*, evil is punished at the end: Quilp drowns, with the waters toying and sporting with the "ghastly freight", much as Quilp had cruelly toyed with his victims.

The Old Curiosity Shop also makes mention of Quilp's physical opposite. Having fled London, Nell and her grandfather meet the travelling players, Codlin and Short. They stop for the night at the Jolly Sandboys public house, where they meet others headed for the same fair. "One of these was the proprietor of a giant." Dickens gives a good presentation of the exploitation of both giants and dwarfs and how they were regarded mostly in terms of market value at exhibitions. This is reflected in *OCS*, Chapter 6, when Kit says that Quilp is "an uglier dwarf than can be seen anywheres for a penny."[49]

The second case of achondroplasia is Miss Mowcher in *David Copperfield*. She is

> a pursy dwarf, of about forty or forty-five, with a very large head and face, a pair of roguish grey eyes ... and though she terminated, as human beings generally do, in a pair of feet, she was so short that she stood at a common-sized chair as at a table (*DC*, 266).

In spite of Dickens's awareness of the exploitation, the use of a dwarf for the person of Miss Mowcher brought a reaction he had not expected. Jane Seymour Hill, a manicurist and chiropodist who lived near Dickens's home, wrote on December 18, 1849 to complain that "All know you have drawn my Portrait." She objected most strongly to Miss Mowcher's role in the seduction of Emily, saying that she had "suffered long and much from [her] personal deformities but never before at the hands of a Man so highly gifted as Charles Dickens and hitherto considered as a Christian and Friend of his fellow Creatures."[50]

This letter (and the threat of litigation) resulted in the promise to change the character, which was done as soon as the story and publication permitted. Dickens wrote to Mrs Hill, apologizing for causing her "unforeseen distress." He went on to make good his promise, turning Miss Mowcher into a heroine. In 1998, Dr James Gamble pointed out that

> Dickens had fallen into the trap of playing to the public image of people with short stature as clowns, freaks, or villains. ... Mrs Jane Seymour Hill's letter made him aware of his own unconscious prejudice, . . . Charles Dickens, the social reformer who was acutely aware of Victorian social ills, took the opportunity to have Miss Mowcher educate the public and put people of short stature in a better light.[51]

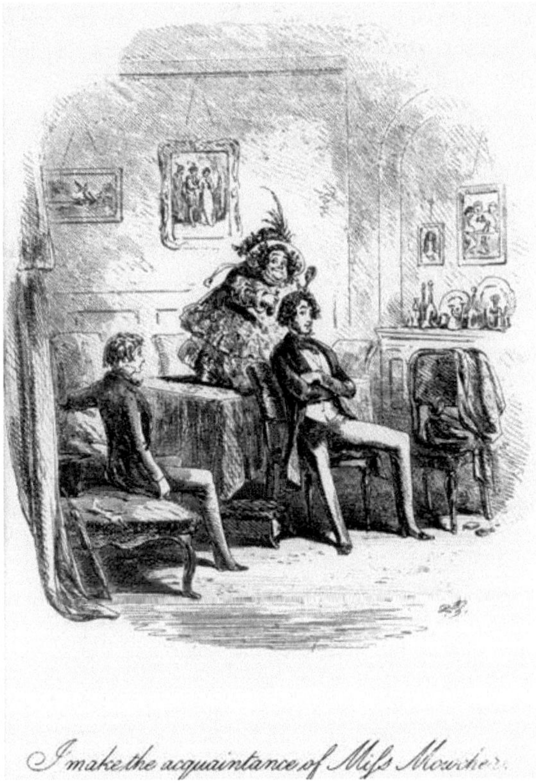

Fig. 4: "I Make the Acquaintance of Miss Mowcher." *David Copperfield.* The Dickens Museum.

Erysipelas

Erysipelas is an acute infection of the skin and subcutaneous tissues caused by group A streptococci.[52] Since bacteriology stems from the late nineteenth century, Dickens could not have known of its genesis; but he definitely knew the appearance of what was termed erysipelas in his day, that it tended to recur, and the folk-medicine term for the disease. According to a nineteenth-century medical dictionary, the term designated "any surface inflammation of the skin with diffuse, not discrete spread" of which there are many forms, with facial erysipelas most common.[53]

The first report of erysipelas in Dickens's works is in *Nicholas Nickleby,* Chapter 44. Sir Mulberry Hawk, injured in an accident caused by Nicholas in defending his sister Kate, is laid up with broken bones and contusions. It is then reported that he has left England and gone to France because of the "danger of another attack of erysipelas – a worse attack – in the head" (*NN,* 568). Interestingly, a medical history book of 1882 cites erysipelas as "most frequently caused by injury."[54]

Perhaps indicating its prevalence, erysipelas is mentioned, but not in a character, in *The Old Curiosity Shop.* Kit Nubbles is arrested for stealing and his mother visits him in jail. The turnkey is not particularly sympathetic and tells Mrs Nubbles that "[Kit] an't the only one in the same fix. You mustn't make a noise about it!" The text goes on:

> With that, he went on reading. The man was not naturally cruel or hard-hearted. He had come to look upon felony as a kind of disorder, like the scarlet fever or erysipelas: some people had it – some hadn't – just as it might be (*OCS*, 473).

The second character with erysipelas is found in Chapter 32 of *Martin Chuzzlewit* (1844):

> Mr Bailey was gone, and had been succeeded (such is the decay of human greatness!) by an old woman whose name was reported to be Tamaroo: which seemed an impossibility. Indeed it appeared in the fulness of time that the jocular boarders had appropriated the word from an English ballad, in which it is supposed to express the bold and fiery nature of a certain hackney-coachman; and that it was bestowed upon Mr Bailey's successor by reason of her having nothing fiery about her, except an occasional attack of that fire which is called St. Anthony's (*MC*, 506).

According to the medical historian Anne Hardy, the name "St. Anthony's fire" refers either to Anthony the Great (third century) or to St. Anthony of Padua (* late twelfth century). Hardy writes that the "fire refers to painful skin infections . . . quite possibly erysipelas or other bacterial skin infections."[55]

The biographer Peter Ackroyd reports that Dickens himself possibly suffered an attack of erysipelas. He was suffering from a "swollen and painful left foot" for which he consulted Sir Henry Thompson. According to Ackroyd, Thompson diagnosed "erysipelas ...consequent upon walking, which might be classed as yet another example of a doctor telling the patient precisely what the patient most wants to hear,"[56] since Dickens apparently was suffering from gout. This version contradicts in part what Forster reported. In August 1867, Thompson apparently let Dickens console himself with the thought that the "enlargement" was "in the nature of a bunion", but erysipelas had "supervened upon the injury".[57] This does not mean that Thompson ascribed the complaint itself to erysipelas. Apparently Thompson was more direct later: in February 1868; Dickens had to cancel a reading due to an "inflammation of the foot (caused by over-exertion)." When the foot was better, he travelled to Scotland, but he found it necessary to consult a medical man there and reported to Forster.

'What made Thompson think it was gout?' [Syme[58]] said often, and seemed to take that opinion extremely ill. Again before leaving Scotland he saw Mr Syme, and wrote to me [Forster] on the second of March of the indignation with which [Syme] again treated the gout diagnosis, declaring the disorder to be an affection of the delicate nerves and muscles originating in cold.[59]

Dickens's apparent self-delusion in this instance has some support in medical texts. The medical dictionary cited above, for example, states that erysipelas in the extremities most often affects the feet and is found especially in people who stand a lot,[60] and *The Lancet of* 1838-39 reports some "Essays in Surgery" by J.M. Coley, Senior Surgeon to Bridgnorth and South Salop Infirmary. Here we find the following concerning erysipelas:

As the cause of the malady as been almost exclusively referred to external injury or irritation, as a lacerated wound … it may not be uninteresting to adduce facts to prove that it may be occasioned by cold.[61]

Gout

What role Dickens's perception of gout as an "aristocratic disease" and his aversion to the aristocracy played in his vehement denial can only be speculated. The signals become blurred, as a review of his gouty characters reveals. Since Dickens was known to eat and drink in moderation,[62] he may simply have rejected a diagnosis rooted in overindulgence.

Considering the eating and drinking habits of upper-middle and upper classes, we might expect a fair number of Dickens's characters to suffer from gout. One limitation might arise from the fact that Dickens more often portrayed people of the lower-middle class and even the lowest class and such people are not apt to suffer from a surfeit of food and drink.

The gouty old aristocrat has been a figure to poke fun at since well before Dickens's day. One of Dickens's favourite authors, Tobias Smollett, has Matthew Bramble of *Humphrey Clinker* say in his first letter to Dr Lewis that "A ridiculous incident … has disordered me in such a manner, that I expect to be laid up with another fit of the gout."[63] The historian Roy Porter points out that *Humphrey Clinker* is "the last novel in any language to select the gouty old man as its hero" and that Smollett included "every socio-economic feature of the topology, proving the joke in the podagra conceit: that they who have been well born pay for it."[64]

Dickens does not remain entirely true to the caricature figure, but mixes classes among the sufferers. The first Dickensian gout victim is the coachman, Tony Weller, in *The Pickwick Papers*. In giving an account of the characters after the close of the narrative, Dickens mentions that Tony "being afflicted with the gout, was compelled to retire" (718). Weller's second wife was the landlady of the "Marquis of Gransby" in Dorking; so his alcohol and food consumption may have been above the norm for his class and thus explain his gout.

Much more in keeping with the traditional aristocratic associations of gout as used by Smollett, the second sufferer is Sir Leicester Dedlock in *Bleak House.* The first presentation of Sir Leicester in Chapter 2 tells us that "his family is as old as the hills, and infinitely more respectable." To identify him further for his contemporary readers, Dickens gives Sir Leicester "a twist of gout now and then." The gouty aristocrat, "deadlocked" in tradition, is more fully described in Chapter 16:

> … his other faithful ally, for better and for worse – the gout – darts into the old oak bed-chamber at Chesney Wold, and grips him by both legs.
>
> Sir Leicester receives the gout as a troublesome demon . . . All the Dedlocks, in the direct male line . . . have had the gout. . . . Other men's fathers may have died of the rheumatism, or may have taken base contagion from the tainted blood of the sick vulgar, but the Dedlock family have communicated something exclusive, even to the leveling process of dying, by dying of their own family gout. . . . Hence, Sir Leicester yields up his family legs to the family disorder. (*BH*, 200-201).

The placement of this description in the novel is interesting. The chapter is headed "Tom-all-Alone's" with reference to a London slum, where we would certainly not expect to find reference to Sir Leicester. But one of the many contrasts in the novel is between the Dedlock's "place in Lincolnshire" and the London slum, and we note the phrase "may have taken base contagion from the tainted blood of the sick vulgar". Here is the contrast in a different form: Sir Leicester suffers the "podagra conceit of the well-born", as Roy Porter put it, while the "sick vulgar" in the novel are represented by Jo, the crossing sweeper, who lives in Tom-all-Alone's. He is the carrier of the base contagion, smallpox, from the London slums to St. Alban's, where the contagion is taken in turn by Lady Dedlock's illegitimate child, Esther Summerson.[65]

Whether Sir Leicester dies as "duty bound" remains unsolved, since he is still alive at the end of the novel. Gout served Dickens in this case as one means of identifying the character type in a way readily recognizable for his contemporary readers. Of particular interest here is the fact that Dickens was aware of the hereditary aspect of gout and could make use of it in his pattern of contrasts.

Continuing in the same vein, the first of two gout victims in *Little Dorrit* (1857) is an aristocrat in the "service" of the State, that is in the Circumlocution Office. When Clennam first goes there to see if he can get any information about

William Dorrit, Barnacle Jr. tells him that his father, Sir Tite Barnacle, has "a slight touch of the gout, and is kept at home by it" (*LD*, 104). Calling on that gentleman, he finds him "in the drawing-room, with his leg on a rest ... the express image of How not to do it" (*LD*, 106). *Bleak House* had used the Court of Chancery as an instrument of satire and the great spider's web in which everyone was caught. *Little Dorrit* has the Circumlocution Office as the epitome of governmental inefficiency and waste. Sir Leicester married into a Chancery case and was not to blame directly, though Dickens does point out the responsibility of people of means towards people of no means, and the speaking name underlines Sir Leicester's resistance to change and reform. But Sir Tite Barnacle is really a cog in the machinery, one of many members of his family who are parasites instead of being the public servants they are paid to be. His "podagra conceit" is apparently both identification and retribution.

The second gout victim in *Little Dorrit* is already dead before the novel begins. Just as Sir Leicester Dedlock expected to die of the family gout, this is one case of gout with fatal outcome, but in a wine-merchant. Flora Finching tells Amy Dorrit that on her honeymoon to Calais "Mr F was in good spirits his appetite was good he liked the cookery he considered the wine weak but palatable and all was well . . ." but that a short time later "Gout flying upwards soared with Mr F to another sphere" (*LD*, 278). Dickens obviously knew of the association between gout and alcohol.

Head Injury

The final two completed novels, *Great Expectations* and *Our Mutual Friend*, each bring a case of cranial trauma. Dickens's clinical observations here are meticulous and convincing, which is especially remarkable considering that the Parisian physician/anthropologist Paul Broca (1824-1880) was just publishing his pioneering research into the localisation of brain functions in 1861, when *Great Expectations* was written.

In *Great Expectations*, Pip's sister is struck down from behind by Orlick. The effects which followed include deafness, double vision, impaired memory, general tremulousness and speech impairment and are plausible from injuries sustained as described:

> Long after . . . my sister lay very ill in bed. Her sight was disturbed, so that she saw objects multiplied . . . her hearing was greatly impaired; her memory also; and her speech was unintelligible . . . A tremulous uncertainty of the action of all her limbs soon became part of her regular state . . . (*GE*, 98).

Our Mutual Friend tells of a murderous attack by the schoolmaster, Bradley Headstone, on his rival, Eugene Wrayburn. Dickens's description of the state two days after the attack is "a remarkable description of the state of fluctuating consciousness which characteristically follows a severe head injury."[66]

> Sometimes his eyes were open, sometimes closed. When they were open, there was no meaning in their unwinking stare at one spot straight before them, unless for a moment the brow knitted into a faint expression of anger, or surprise. Then, Mortimer Lightwood would speak to him, and on occasions he would be so far roused as to make an attempt to pronounce his friend's name. But, in an instant consciousness was gone again, and no spirit of Eugene was in Eugene's crushed outer form (*OMF*, 805-6).

The attack is the oft-encountered literary trope of near-death/moral rebirth. Eugene, barely surviving – and that thanks only to Lizzie Hexham, who pulled him out of the river – finally has some direction in life.

Injuries resulting in unexpected debility

The scene in *Nicholas Nickleby* describing injuries resulting from a beating is simply too funny to be omitted, though it has nothing whatever to do with serious medicine. Nicholas, enraged beyond endurance by Squeers's abuse of Smike, beats the schoolmaster and returns to London. Squeers's daughter, Fanny, writes to Nicholas's uncle, Ralph:

> My pa requests me to write to you, the doctors considering it doubtful whether he will ever recuvver the use of his legs which prevents his holding a pen (*NN*, 175).

The letter continues in this vein and is so very ludicrous that one is surprised to find the same device used by Mrs Gaskell in *Cranford*, originally published in *Household Words* beginning in December 1851. In Chapter 5 "Old Letters", we read:

> His wife (Miss Jenkyns's grandmother) did not write, said the old gentleman, because he had forbidden it, she being indisposed with a sprained ankle, which (he said) quite incapacitated her from holding a pen.[67]

Malaria

Malaria is one of the diseases described by Dickens which, in Dr John Cosnett's view, "warrant no debate".[68] In the American segment of *Martin Chuzzlewit*, both young Martin and Mark Tapley contract malaria in Eden, a "hideous swamp choked with slime and matted growth, where fatal maladies … came forth at night, in misty shapes, and creeping upon the water, hunted them like spectres until day" (*MC*, 375).

The description of the attack corresponds to the initial "cold" stage of the disease, which lasts from 20 to 60 minutes:[69]

> They found Martin in the house, lying wrapped up in his blanket on the ground. He was, to all appearances, very ill indeed, and shook and shivered horribly; not as people do from cold, but in a frightful kind of spasm or convulsion, that racked his whole body (*MC*, 517).

Sir Patrick Manson (1844-1922) first proposed his malaria-mosquito theory in 1879, which was confirmed in 1894 in cooperation with Sir Ronald Ross (1857-1932). But the disease has been known since antiquity and was considered among the "miasmal" diseases. The term malaria, from the Italian "mala" and "aria" ("bad air") was in use in Italy by the seventeenth century to refer to the cause of intermittent fevers from exposure to marsh air or miasma. Horace Walpole wrote in 1740 about a "horrid thing called mal'aria". This may have been the first appearance of the term in print. But Walpole meant the presumed cause; the shift in meaning from the cause to the disease itself occurred in the late nineteenth century, when the causative agents were identified.[70] Not long before Dickens wrote *Chuzzlewit, The Lancet* reported on a meeting of the Westminster Medical Society. One of the members, Dr Addison, made some observations on malaria.

> In the first place, what did we mean by the term malaria? The original meaning of the word was simply "bad air"; this however, did not exactly express that which he wished to bring under discussion. He should, therefore, define it to be a something recognized chiefly by its effects on the general health, and occurring in certain localities, under certain circumstances, for the evolution of this something the presence of moisture, a certain degree of temperature, and vegetable matter, being required. He distinguished malaria, as thus defined, entirely from that influence by which plague, small-pox, and other contagious diseases were propagated.[71]

Another Society member, Dr A Thomson, commented that he "had no doubt but that malaria was a gas, but of its nature we were completely ignorant."

It is interesting to note that when he went to the United States for the second time, Dickens's travelling medicine chest included quinine, probably as an anti-malarial. Malaria – as Dickens well knew – was endemic on the North American continent.[72]

While malaria has largely been brought under control in developed countries - even in "Eden" – it remains a major health problem, especially in sub-Saharan Africa, where between 300 and 500 million people contract malaria and more than 1 million die each year.[73]

Marfan Syndrome

One character has been identified as suffering from Marfan Syndrome, the most conspicuous external features of which are the disproportion between the upper and lower body segments, excessively long finger bones and an arm span which may exceed body height.[74] Dr John Cosnett has apparently based the identification simply on there being "too much lengthwise and not enough sidewise" of the young man, Sloppy, in *Our Mutual Friend.*[75] If Cosnett's assumption is correct, this would be another instance of Dickens's observations preceding those of the medical profession. The syndrome was identified in 1894 by the French paediatrician Jean-Bernard-Antoine Marfan (1858-1942). According to *Harrison's*, Marfan Syndrome has a prevalence of "more than 1 in 50,000, perhaps 1 in 10,000." While Marfan Syndrome may apply to Sloppy, the clinical information (dislocated lens, aortic dilatation) on which a definitive diagnosis could be based is missing; Sloppy may just have been tall; he was likely undernourished and thus thin, even if otherwise healthy.

Measles-Pneumonia

Johnny, the orphan who is to be adopted by the Boffins in *Our Mutual Friend,* contracts a contagious disease, apparently from two other small children cared for by Johnny's grandmother, Betty Higden. Sloppy, who reports the illness to John Rokesmith, can only report that

> 'they come out upon him and partickler his chest ... there was some of 'em wot you couldn't kiver with a sixpence.' Pressed to fall back upon a nominative case, he opined that they wos about as red as ever red could be. 'But as long as they strikes out'ards, sir... they ain't so much. It's their striking in'ards that's to be kep off' (*OMF*, 378).

Sloppy also says that Johnny complained of "choking," so the child likely had contracted measles with a superimposed pulmonary infection. He is taken to a hospital – apparently the Great Ormond Street Hospital for Sick Children – where the doctor says it is "too late" and the child dies. This is not criticism of the hospital, however, but rather a plea that parents take their sick children to the hospital *before* it's too late.

The medical historian Anne Hardy reports that measles was one of the major killers of children under 5 in the nineteenth century. "Under adverse social conditions . . . bronchitis and broncho-pneumonia are damaging (and the latter often fatal) sequelae."[76]

Metabolic Disorder

One rather grotesque character found in *Little Dorrit* is Maggy, who is

> about eight-and-twenty, . . . with large feet and hands, large eyes and no hair. Her large eyes were limpid and almost colorless; they seemed to be very little affected by light, and to stand unnaturally still. There was also that attentive listening expression in her face, which is seen in the faces of the blind; but she was not blind, having one tolerably serviceable eye (*LD*, 96/7).

In this prison novel, Maggy's form of imprisonment is mental retardation, which Amy Dorrit attributes to her having had a bad fever at the age of ten and never maturing beyond that point. Lord Brain postulates that the disease may have been meningitis or encephalitis, which, he says "might be inferred on general grounds." He goes on to quote the above description and asks: "Was this the first account of what came to be known as the Argyll-Robertson pupil?"[77] He leaves the question unanswered, however.

More recently, Howard Markel suggested that Maggy may have had phenylketonuria.[78] This error in the metabolism of an essential amino acid was first described in 1934 and would explain Maggy's "limpid, colorless eyes," since the body is incapable of producing dark pigments. The condition can also result in mental retardation. Modern treatment consists mainly of a low phenylalanine diet. Maggy's diet likely consisted of bread, milk, green vegetables, potatoes and cheese, and thus contained enough protein to exacerbate the condition. She is also very fond of "chicking," another high source of phenylalanine.

This condition would not explain Maggy's large features and extremities. Dickens may simply have used Maggy's largeness and physique in contrast to her mental handicap. Since the eponymous heroine of this novel is "Little Dorrit" and she is the only one in her family who is mature in any real sense of the word, Maggy's size may also be in contrast to her "Little Mother."

Paget's Disease

In *Martin Chuzzlewit*, when young Martin and Mark Tapley return to England, they go to the Blue Dragon in the village where Pecksniff lives. Among other people, they see the tailor, who in Mark's description, is

> a little bandyer than he was. . . . His figure's so far altered . . . that you might wheel a rather larger barrow between his legs as he walks, than you could have done conweniently when we know'd him (*MC*, 656).

Dr John Cosnett writes that the tailor "must have had Paget's Disease of bone,"[79] which was first described by the English surgeon and pathologist Sir James Paget (1814-1899) in 1877, 33 years after publication of *Martin Chuzzlewit.* Paget's disease is nothing new: it was suspected in a Neanderthal skull. Its uniqueness lies in that it only affects adult humans (males more than females by a ratio of 3:2).[80] The cause of the disease remains unclear, but one characteristic cited by *Harrison's* is a "lateral bowing of the femur,"[81] which is obviously the tailor's problem.

Paralysis

Some form of paralysis is observed in several characters, but in at least two of these, its origin is psychosomatic. Since psychosomatic medicine is omitted from this study, they would not be included here had Lord Brain not mentioned these characters and expressed some doubt concerning them. The first of the two is Tommy Traddles's mother-in-law in *David Copperfield.* Mrs Crewler, wrote Lord Brain, "was … a paraplegic, but there is a good deal of evidence that her paraplegia was hysterical."[82] Actually there is no evidence of the origin of the underlying disorder; it may in fact have been physical. Traddles tells David:

> [S]he is a very superior woman, but has lost the use of her limbs. *Whatever occurs to harass her usually settles in her legs*; but on this occasion (of Traddles and Sophy announcing their engagement), it … pervaded the whole system in a most alarming manner. However, *they brought her through it by unremitting and affectionate attention* (*DC*, 675; my emphasis).

Mrs Crewler obviously used her affliction as an instrument of blackmail whenever her family threatened to overlook her and pay attention to anyone else, but this does not preclude an actual physical crippling.

The second "hysterical paralytic" is Mrs Clennam in *Little Dorrit.* Lord Brain says she is harder to diagnose, since she spent her life on a sofa, but "astonished everybody toward the end of the novel by suddenly getting up and rushing out of the house."[83] It is possible that, like Miss Havisham in *Great Expectations,* who was never seen eating, Mrs Clennam walked about at night when nobody was around to see her. She did, in any event, get up from her chair, and after tottering just a few steps, run through the city to prevent Arthur's learning the truth of his birth; so she had more muscle tone than would have been expected.

Jane Wood, discussing Mrs Clennam in conjunction with "the medicalization of womanhood" points out that Mrs Clennam's emotional repression has "turned into a self-consuming mental malady which mimics consumptive disease."[84] While physical crippling is associated with certain forms of tuberculosis, it is not necessarily part of phthisis. As discussed in Chapter 5, the "consumptive" or "fading" form of tuberculosis is portrayed quite differently by Dickens than his portrayal of the forceful personality of Mrs Clennam. Certainly no nineteenth-century reader would have associated Mrs Clennam with consumption. Her paralysis, however, since it is clearly self-imposed and not due to physical causes, is not discussed here. For the purposes of this study, Mrs Clennam is uninteresting until she has a stroke and she is discussed in that connection in Chapter 4.

A true case of paraplegia is represented by Grandfather Smallweed in *Bleak House*: "He is in a helpless condition as to his lower, and nearly so as to his upper limbs; but his mind is unimpaired" (*BH*, 264). He is a mean, spiteful, avaricious old man who must be propped up by his granddaughter whenever he sinks down in his chair, usually because he has thrown a cushion at his wife, who suffers senile dementia. No physical details are given as to the cause of paralysis, and the use appears to be metaphorical in connection with the crippling effects of overweening love of money.

Pneumonia

Pneumonia, like so many diseases in the nineteenth century, was practically untreatable and thus even more life-threatening than in our time. It was considered "the most frequent of the inflammatory diseases, which spares no age group." [85] Dick Swiveller in *The Old Curiosity Shop* starts out as a less-than-admirable character. He is frequently inebriated, does as little work as he can and initially joins Fred Trent's plot against Little Nell. Dickens uses the trope of illness/near death to convert Dick into a better human being.

> But the lives of gentlemen devoted to such pleasures as Richard Swiveller, are extremely precarious. The spiritual excitement of the last fortnight, working upon a system affected in no slight degree by the spirituous excitement of some years, proved a little too much for him. That very night, Mr Richard was seized with an alarming illness, and in twenty-four hours was stricken with a raging fever (*OCS*, 490).

When Swiveller finally awakes out of delirium, he finds the Marchioness tending him and that he had been ill to the point of death for nearly three weeks. R.T. Young, writing in the *Cornhill Magazine* in 1934 "diagnoses" the case as pneumonia:

> Dick Swiveller is down with pneumonia in his one shabby lodging-room. No doctor is called, no nurse installed (not a professional one at any rate), no removal to hospital is suggested. . . . [B]ut for [The Marchioness's] care, Dick would very likely have died. And after all, she has done not badly by making him as clean and comfortable as she can, and just letting him lie till the "crisis" has come.[86]

The diagnosis is plausible. *Harrison's* cites a form of pneumonia in which the "first symptoms of myalgia and headache are followed by fever, chills and a cough" and "confusion or delirium are common."[87] There is also a connection made to alcohol abuse in connection with lowered resistance to the pathogens causing pneumonia. Young's statement that no doctor is called in is, however, incorrect: the Marchioness tells Dick that "the doctor had left word he might refresh himself when he awoke" (*OCS*, 494) and also that Dick "was to be kept quite still, and there was to be no noise nor nothing" (*OCS*, 496).

Dick learns from the Marchioness how Kit Nubbles had been framed and manages from his sick bed to direct Kit's exoneration, in his first act of selfless maturity.

Pulmonary Obstruction

Two characters appear to suffer from pulmonary obstruction. The first is Major Bagstock in *Dombey and Son*, who is generally referred to as "the blue-faced major." He considers himself above everyone and

> "... tough, Sir, tough, and de-vilish sly!" After such a declaration, wheezing sounds would be heard; and the Major's blue would deepen into purple, while his eyes strained and started convulsively (*DS*, 92).

The wheezing and colour are used to identify the Major. A medical dictionary of 1842[88] cites dyspnea and wet cough, facial colour tending to purple, with purple and swollen lips as typical of emphysema, and this "diagnosis" is found in a medical review of this character: Lord Brain refers to the Major "with his lobster eyes and horse's cough, panting, blowing and gasping with his bronchitis and emphysema."[89]

The second character is the turnkey, Bob, at the Marshalsea Prison, where William Dorrit is imprisoned for debt and "Little Dorrit" is born. In 1930, Dr Dwight O'Hara wrote in the *New England Journal of Medicine:*

> There may be, as affirmed in a late statement from the Massachusetts General Hospital, no such thing as emphysema, but we have all seen men go down, as the turnkey who died on the lock of the Marshalsea prison:
>
> 'Time went on, and the turnkey began to fail. His chest swelled, and his legs got weak, and he was short of breath. ... He sat in an arm-chair with a cushion, and sometimes wheezed so, for minutes together, that he couldn't turn the key' (*LD, 65).*[90]

Renal Colic

Dickens reported suffering severe pain in his left side, which he ascribed to an inflamed kidney.[91] No diagnosis is known; speculation runs from renal colic, kidney stones even to renal tuberculosis. Whatever it was, Dickens seems to have described it in old Martin Chuzzlewit:

> Here was the old gentlemen, who had taken this step [staying on at the Blue Dragon] by reason of his sudden illness in the carriage, suffering the most horrible cramps and spasms, yet protesting and vowing in the midst of his pain, that he wouldn't have a doctor sent for, and wouldn't take any remedies but those which the young lady administered from a small medicine chest. . . . (*MC*, 26).

Mary Graham, in response to Mrs Lupin's saying "what a Providence" it was that she had the medications on hand, reported that "they are intended for such an emergency. We never travel without them" (*MC*, 28). So old Martin's suffering was periodic, like Dickens's, and could be relieved by specific remedies. Dickens's travelling medicine chest contained a quantity of opiates, such as laudanum, "the aspirin of its day because it was one of only few drugs that brought relief in a variety of conditions."[92]

"Sleep apnea"

Sleep apnea or the "sleep-induced apnea syndrome" is a term not coined until 1972.[93] An article by Dr Meir Kryger entitled "Sleep Apnea" was cited above in the discussion of the Pickwickian Syndrome. The only Dickensian character Dr Kryger discusses is Joe, but he does mention Pickwick himself, saying:

> Samuel Pickwick, the obese hero of the piece, did not have sleep apnea – except perhaps when intoxicated: 'The wine ... had exerted its somniferous influence . . . upon the senses of Mr Pickwick. . . . His head was sunk upon his bosom; and perpetual snoring, with a partial choke occasionally, were the only audible indications of this great man's presence.'[94]

In his article "Fat, Sleep and Charles Dickens" published three years later, Kryger enlarges on this, pointing out that "only very recently has it been reported in the medical literature that alcohol can induce apnea during sleep in otherwise normal people."[95]

Dr John Cosnett appears to be of a different opinion than Kryger. He points out that the term "Pickwickian Syndrome" is sometimes applied to what is today known as the "sleep apnea syndrome," but places obstructive sleep apnea apart. The figure he cites in this connection is John Willet, proprietor of the Maypole Inn in *Barnaby Rudge*. Willet "began to doze . . . his breathing was pretty much the same . . . save that he sometimes experienced a slight difficulty in respiration (such as a carpenter meets with when he is planing and comes to a knot)" (*BR*, 316). Later Willet had "got into such a complication of knots, that it was perfectly clear he must wake or die. He chose the former alternative, and opened his eyes" (*BR*, 317). "Dickens," says Cosnett, "seems to have realized the potential mortality of obstructive sleep apnea."[96]

Considering the controversy surrounding the Pickwick syndrome, what it is or isn't and its connection with sleep apnea, it is interesting to note that Dickens obviously separated the two. *Barnaby Rudge* was completed only five years after *Pickwick* and the totally different use of the two states is conspicuous. John Willet has, of course, a different role with a plausibly much more serious purpose than the fat boy. Since Willet also suffers a stroke, he is discussed in that connection in Chapter 4.

Sleep Paralysis

Oliver Twist, brings another state which is open to several possible interpretations. This is the scene in Chapter 37 in which Oliver, at the Maylie's, falls asleep over his books and "sees" Fagin and Monks looking in the window of the room.

> There is a kind of sleep that steals upon us sometimes, which, while it holds the body prisoner, does not free the mind from a sense of things about it, and enable it to ramble at its pleasure. . . . It is an undoubted fact, that although our senses of touch and sight be for the time dead, yet our sleeping thoughts, and the visionary scenes that pass before us, will be influenced, and materially influenced, by the *mere silent presence* of some external object: which may not have been near us when we closed our eyes: and of whose vicinity we have had no waking consciousness (*OT*, 227-8).

Oliver, in this state, "hears" Fagin talking to another man, whom he recognizes as the stranger who had accosted him earlier. On Oliver's raising the alarm about seeing the two men, a search is instituted, but not even footprints can be found.

Dennis Walder in *Dickens and Religion* has proffered a religious explanation of a "trance-like moment of recognition between good and evil," [97] while Fred Kaplan is of the opinion that this is one of the many mesmeric episodes to be found in Dickens's works. [98] This is supported by Alison Winter who hypothesizes in *Mesmerized* that due to the high interest in "animal magnetism" at the time the novel was written, Dickens's contemporaries would have "had no difficulty in diagnosing this state as magnetic." [99] Winter's argument is weakened by speaking of Oliver's "ability to see events occurring miles away." While Fagin and Monks were undoubtedly in London, Oliver "saw" them looking in the window of the room where he sat. It appears more likely to me that Oliver had the not uncommon experience of a bad dream in which two people who frightened him, but who to his knowledge were completely unconnected, appeared as a threat to the safe surroundings in which he then found himself.

One opinion has been expressed from a medical point of view, which is more germane to the present discussion. Dr John Cosnett quotes the above passage, saying that it makes clear "[t]hat Dickens was aware of the phenomenon of sleep paralysis." He goes on to point out that sleep paralysis was first described by Weir Mitchell in 1876, nearly 40 years after publication of *Oliver Twist*. [100]

Tourette's Syndrome

One of the many characters who is identified by physical characteristics is the rent collector, Pancks, in *Little Dorrit*. He "snorted and sniffed and puffed and blew, like a little labouring steam engine" and is likened to a dingy little steam-tug (*LD*, 143-4). The simile sometimes appears a little overdone, but it is likely that Dickens had observed a person with Tourette's Syndrome. This syndrome, first described by the French physician, George Gilles de la Tourette (1857-1904) in 1885, about thirty years after publication of *Little Dorrit*, [101] is characterized, among other things, by grimaces, barking, coughing and muscular tics. Many patients also show obsessive-compulsive behavior – in Pancks's case, collecting and recording information in his note-book:

> In his tracking out of the claim to its complete establishment, Mr Pancks had shown a sagacity that nothing could baffle, and a patience and secresy that nothing could tire (*LD*, 399).

Pancks's perseverance resulted in William Dorrit's release from prison after a quarter of a century of incarceration for another man's debt.

Typhoid

One case of typhoid appears in a Dickens novel. [102] Sairey Gamp, already hired to take care of Chuffey, Anthony Chuzzlewit's old clerk, approaches the undertaker, Mr Mould, about taking on an additional job.

> There *is* a gent, sir, at the Bull in Holborn, as has been took ill there, and is bad abed. They have a day nurse as was recommended from Bartholomew's … But she is otherways engaged at night, and they are in wants of night-watching (*MC*, 405/6).

Mr Mould agrees to her taking the job from eight to eight, and she goes off to the inn. Arriving there, she hears John Westlock and the landlord discussing the patient. John says:

> [A]s the medical man says the fever must take its course, and nothing can be done just now beyond giving him his drinks regularly and having him carefully attended to, nothing more can be said that I know of, until he is in a condition to give us some information (*MC*, 408).

In 1934, R.T.Young stressed the difference between his time and Dickens's day, one of the greatest differences being this scene at the Bull:

> The contrast between Dickens's day and our own is . . . strikingly emphasised in the case of Lewsome (*Martin Chuzzlewit*). Not even the first beginnings of the science of Public Health are discernible. Lewsome, suffering from typhoid, is allowed to lie for weeks *in a hotel*, a thing unthinkable today. [103]

Young's diagnosis would appear supported by a statement by Pierre Louis (1787-1872) of Paris, who held, after statistical comparison of various treatments, that the course of typhoid fever could neither be interrupted nor shortened by treatment, and that the physician ought to depend mainly on the healing power of nature. Louis was, however, convinced that typhoid and typhus were identical. Louis's student, the US physician William Wood Gerhard (1809-1872), first distinguished between the two, although his evidence was not immediately accepted. The final recognition was brought by the work of William Jenner (1815-1898) at the London Fever Hospital.[104]

Wry Neck

Jeremiah Flintwinch, in *Little Dorrit,* is another character identified by a morbid condition. His "head was awry" (*LD,* 33) and "his neck so twisted that the knotted ends of his white cravat usually dangled under one ear" (*LD,* 37). Dr Cosnett writes that "this can only have been a case of focal dystonia with torticollis" and points out that Dickens observed a feature "which might only be in small print in medical texts: Flintwinch is noted, on several occasions, to 'scrape his horny cheek'. This is the *geste antagoniste*, which relieves the disorder by counter-pressure".[105]

Conclusion

There are many "clinical miniatures", as Lord Brain called them, in Dickens's works. Here we have found confirmation of the talent for observation and facility of description cited by the writer of Dickens's obituary in the *British Medical Journal* (see Chapter 1). Dickens described a multitude of medical entities, several in advance of their perception by the profession. While research and medical instrumentation have led to further elucidation of these entities, they have – astoundingly – not led to rejection or correction of Dickens's descriptions.

This survey has included only the physical states and disabilities and not even all of those. To include all cases of crippling, artificial limbs, childhood diseases, or use of medical terms in non-medical settings would undoubtedly more than double the length of this chapter without adding substantially to our knowledge. Instead, we now turn our attention to four specific diseases which play a larger role in Dickens's works. The discussion starts with disorders afflicting individual sufferers and proceeds to epidemic diseases which were sociomedical issues in their own right in the nineteenth century. We begin with epilepsy or epileptiform seizures, which can be identified in six of Dickens's characters.

---

[1] Cosnett (2003), 27.
[2] Bethel (1970) 25.
[3] MacDonald Critchley (1900-1997) defined a "Miss Havisham Syndrome" in psychiatry in 1969.
[4] *Dickensian*, 1-2, 9-13, here 10-11; original italics.
[5] Fothergill, cited in Kryger, (1985) 560.
[6] W. Wadd. *Cursory Remarks on Corpulence*. Cited in Markel (1985), 24-6.
[7] London (1968), 448-52.
[8] Geisler (1971), 212-216.
[9] Lavie (1984), 2025-28.
[10] Herrmann (1997), 80. My translation.
[11] See Herrmann (1997), 8, 9.
[12] Cosnett. *Sleep* (1992), 266. For a definition of Kleine-Levin Syndrome, see Glossary.
[13] Cosnett. (1997) 201. The variant ways of writing "cardiorespiratory" are in the respective originals.
[14] Cosnett (2003), 26.
[15] In: Herrmann, 85.
[16] Fielding,K.J. (1996), 119-134
[17] Letter from E.J. Collings, President of the Manchester branch of the Dickens Fellowship, to the editor of the *Dickensian*, published in 1-2, 1905-1906, 194. It's astounding that a burglar and murderer was invited to entertain at a school shortly after having shot someone.
[18] Published in London, 1912.
[19] Kryger (1983), 2301.
[20] Stannard, 264.
[21] *Enzyklopaedisches Wörterbuch der medicinischen Wissenschaften [EWmW],* 3 (1829), 575. All entries cited from this work are my translation.
[22] *The Lancet*, II, 1837-38, 97.
[23] In medical experience, patients still report this effect, but whether the effect is pharmacological or psychological is unclear. Alternatively, Mr Omer may have been burning atropine (belladonna) in his pipe, since it was used to treat asthma as early as the Middle Ages. About 1890 (probably earlier), "antiasthma cigarettes" were sold as a cure for "asthma and influenza," containing "no narcotic substance". They contained about 2.4 mg

hyoscyamine, which was converted to atropine on burning. (Atropine is classed as a dangerous drug, but not as a narcotic.) [Wellcome Library network information]
[24] *Harrison' Principles of Internal Medicine,* Ed. 9, 1980, [*Harrison's*] 1203. An article in *The Medical Post* (Canada) of April 8, 2003, reports an increased mortality in asthmatic patients, whereby the patient is 3.5 times more likely to die of chronic obstructive pulmonary disease than non-asthmatic patients. (p. 64).
[25] Jacoby, "Charles Dickens' Asthma" (1995), 34.
[26] *Ibid* 37.
[27] *Ibid,* 38.
[28] *Ibid* 39.
[29] Fowler's term for the "facts only", unimaginative philosophy of the character Thomas Gradgrind.
[30] Fowler. In: Connor (1996), 107/8.
[31] *Letters* 4, 48.
[32] *Ibid*, 79.
[33] Quétel, 134.
[34] The Regency Period in England lasted from 1811 to 1820.
[35] Johann Kaspar Lavater, Swiss theologian, poet and physiognomist.
[36] See, for example, Rawdon Crawley in Thackeray's *Vanity Fair* and Mr Pullett in Eliot's *The Mill on the Floss.*
[37] Tytler, 211.
[38] This typically "Dickensian" description is actually taken from Sheridan's "The Rivals", Act III, Scene I.
[39] Sudoffs Archive, Beiheft 2, 1963, 5-6.
[40] Pahor (1979), 1.
[41] *Ibid*, 2.
[42] *Ibid,* 3.
[43] J. Toynbee. *Diseases of the Ear*, London 1860, 235, 335, 352, 395. in: Pahor, 1.
[44] Markel (1984), 408. Authors disagree whether the first "e" is with or without accent.
[45] Pfaltz and Alford (1986), 3.
[46] Gamble (1998), 9.
[47] Romano, 24.
[48] Wainapel, 632.
[49] A giant, Pickleson, makes an appearance in a traveling caravan in *Marigold.* The exploitation also applies to excessively fat people; see the description of Joe (*PP*) above.
[50] Cited in Gamble (1998), 10.
[51] Gamble (1998), 12.
[52] *Harrison's,* 617.
[53] *EWmW,* 11, (1834), 486.
[54] *Geschichte der Medicin...* (1882), 699.
[55] Hardy in: Kiple (1993), 989-90.
[56] Ackroyd, *Dickens*, 1000-1001.
[57] Forster II, 323.
[58] James Syme (1799-1870) had been Thompson's professor.
[59] Forster II, 445-46.
[60] *EWmW, 486*
[61] *The Lancet*, I, 1838-39, 44.
[62] Johnson, 2, 1054. Claire Tomalin questions this in a review of the most recent volume of Dickens's letters (*TLS*, September 6, 2002), at least with respect to Dickens's alcohol consumption.

[63] Everyman Edition, 7.
[64] Porter and Rousseau. (1998), 94/5. Porter also points out that Wilkie Collins suffered gout before the age of 30, and his correspondence with Dickens remains "one of the great archives in the annals of gout" (173).
[65] See Chapter 6, "Smallpox".
[66] Brain (1955), 134.
[67] Elizabeth Gaskell, *Cranford*, Penguin Edition, 1994, 62.
[68] Cosnett (2003), 24.
[69] Dickens notes that recovery is slow and exhausting, but does not detail the following "hot stage" of fever, and "wet stage" of profuse sweating [*Harrison's*, 870].
[70] Dunn, 861.
[71] *The Lancet*, February 16, 1839, 811.
[72] Dickens and Jacoby, 23.
[73] "Beside malaria, SARS pales as killer" Barry James *International Herald Tribune*, April 26-27, 2003, 2.
[74] *Harrison's*, 532-3.
[75] Cosnett (2003), 26.
[76] Hardy,
[77] Brain (1955), 136.
[78] Markel. *The Dickensian*, 76, 1982, 120-1.
[79] Cosnett (2003), 26.
[80] Altman, 911 and 913.
[81] *Harrison's*, 1861.
[82] Brain (1955), 130.
[83] *Ibid*, 131.
[84] Wood (2001), 44.
[85] *EWmW*. 127, (1842) 685.
[86] Young, 713.
[87] *Harrison's* 1226.
[88] *EWmW*, 10, (1834), 639.
[89] Brain (1960), 145.
[90] O'Hara. (1930), 1083.
[91] Letter to F.M. Evans dated July 3, 1849, for example.
[92] Dickens and Jacoby, *24*.
[93] Herrmann, 83.
[94] Kryger, 1983, 2302.
[95] Kryger, 1985, 558.
[96] Cosnett *(Sleep*, 1992) 267.
[97] London, 1981, Chapter 2, footnote 6.
[98] Kaplan (1975) 130. See also Chapter 8, "mesmerism".
[99] Winter (1998) 58.
[100] Cosnett, (*Sleep, 1992)*, 265.
[101] Cosnett, (1998), 131.
[102] For a description of typhoid and its differentiation from typhus, see Chapter 6 "Smallpox".
[103] Young, 714.
[104] Wilson in Bynum and Porter (1993), 401-403.
[105] Cosnett (1998), 131.

CHAPTER 3: Epilepsy

Epilepsy is one disorder which Dickens uses more than once. The symptom of seizure, for "an epileptic seizure is not a disease but a symptom,"[1] is described as a predominant characteristic of three figures, while epilepti-form seizures appear in two and possibly three others. With epilepsy, as noted generally, Dickens does not specifically name the disorder, and it is interesting to note what term Dickens uses to convey his intention and, by comparison with medical texts, whether his use emphasises his lay status. Also of interest is the history of epilepsy: what was known of its genesis, how were patients viewed, and how were they treated in Dickens's time?

History

"Epilepsy" – or at least a condition characterized by sudden outbreaks of convulsions – has been known and reported since ancient times. Hippocrates (or one of his school) attacked the concept that an epileptic was spirit-possessed, saying that divinity was used "as a pretext and screen of [the physician's] inability to offer any assistance."[2] This recognition did not stop the Gospel writers from accepting a satanic origin of seizures. Epilepsy was even considered contagious – one of eight cardinal contagious diseases, along with bubonic plague, tuberculosis, scabies (a parasitic skin infection), erysipelas (see Chapter 2), anthrax (a highly-infectious animal disease which can be transmitted to humans), trachoma (a Chlamydia parasitic infection) and leprosy. Belief in the contagiousness of convulsions was one reason for social ostracism. It also led to the establishment of special hospitals for epileptics, apart from the insane asylums where epileptics were frequently confined, but more in order to protect the insane from contagion than out of consideration for the epileptics.[3]

In 1770, the Swiss physician Samuel-Auguste Tissot (1728-1797) published a comprehensive treatise on epilepsy or "the falling sickness." According to Temkin, Tissot's book was still widely read in the early nineteenth century,[4] making it a plausible – albeit speculative – source for Dickens. Several points raised by Tissot can be noted among Dickens's apparently epileptic characters, which may support this hypothesis. While it is tempting to think Dickens might have read Tissot's text – it was apparently never translated into English, but Dickens was fluent in French – it is perhaps more likely that he was familiar with a series of lectures published in *The Lancet* which made considerable use of Tissot's work.[5]

Tissot points out that the one characteristic common to seizures is a loss of consciousness, which he considers essential to the diagnosis. This remained the medical opinion until well into the nineteenth century. In an abstract of a clinical lecture by Dr Wilks (Guy's Hospital), published in *The Lancet* of February 26,

1870, it is stated that "loss of consciousness is essential to the definition of epilepsy; convulsions occurring without loss of consciousness are not truly epileptic." This has been superseded by the current classification of seizures into: I. Partial (focal, local) seizures, classified primarily according to whether consciousness is affected or not: in "simple partial" seizures, consciousness is not affected, in "complex partial" it is; II. Generalized seizures (convulsive or non-convulsive). Consciousness may be impaired, and impairment may be the initial manifestation. III. Unclassified epileptic seizures, which "defy classification."[6]

Although much of what was believed in the eighteenth century has now been rejected, several of Tissot's observations have retained their validity. For example, he writes of the spontaneous remission of seizures, and of cranial trauma as a possible cause. He reports on alcohol-related seizures, and on patients able to suppress the onset of seizures. His observations also include a statement that seizures are not uniform, either inter- or intra-patient.

Contributing to the misconceptions about epilepsy, Tissot sees moral and physical causes of the disease. The moral causes are: "violent passions, insults to the soul, overexertion of the mind, and prolonged cogitation."[7] Among the passions, Tissot says that fear is the most common cause, but wrath and worry may also elicit seizures. Licentiousness, as endangering the soul, is a cause, as is studiousness immediately after meals. According to Temkin, "the etiological relevancy of fright and 'moral' causes in general was scarcely as much as doubted."[8]

The question of treatment of epilepsy in the days of rudimentary pharmacology is interesting historically, although its relevance for Dickens is slight, since he describes no treatment. According to Tissot, the ancients had recommended bleeding to "relieve the congestion of the brain". But this was unnecessary in Tissot's opinion, because the patient frequently suffered nosebleeds and bleeding a patient in convulsions was difficult at best. Still, the *Edinburgh Medical Journal* half-a-century later said that

> On the presumption of [epilepsy] depending at least in part, on plethora, many of the most esteemed authors recommend frequent bloodletting, purging, emetics, blisters, [etc.].[9]

It is noted in connection with Anthony Chuzzlewit (see below and also Chapter 4) that the patient was bled – but whether this was due to the epileptiform seizure which preceded his stroke or because of the stroke itself cannot be ascertained.

Terminology

Some of the terms still used to designate certain epileptic attacks have retained their French forms: *grand mal, petit mal* and *absence*. Temkin notes that these terms "do not indicate any form of epilepsy unknown before the nineteenth century."[10] *Le grand mal* is taken to mean a fully-developed fit with loss of consciousness and general convulsions, while *le petit mal* is, in Temkin's words, "badly defined." The current neurological definition of *petit mal* is "a type of seizure (absence seizures) that in contrast to the *grand mal* seizure, are noted for their brevity and for the degree of loss of awareness (brief staring spell) accompanied by minimal motor manifestations."[11] Temkin compares these terms with their medieval analogs, *epilepsia maior* and *epilepsia minor*, which "connotated two stereotyped forms of epileptic fits." But he admits that he is not definitely able to say whether there is "a real historical connection between these two sets of names."[12]

Customarily not naming the morbid state, Dickens does not use any of these terms. It is seen that although the word "seizure" is used in describing Guster in *Bleak House* even that use was unique in Dickens's works. The term he most commonly uses is "fits." However, this term does not emphasise Dickens's lay status, nor was the use of the term limited to the nineteenth century: a case report was published in 1998 by D. Burgner et al. in *The Lancet* saying that a six-year-old boy was "discharged home the next day, to be readmitted 12 hours later with further fits."[13]

Of course, the term is not used exclusively to indicate epilepsy. The chapter on stroke discusses victims of "fits" which were more likely apoplexy or stroke. Various causes of "fits" are found in Dickens's works. The performance of "The Blood-Drinker's Burial" by Miss Petowker in *Nicholas Nickleby* elicited terror in the little Kenwigses, "who were all but frightened into fits" (*NN*, 170). In *The Old Curiosity Shop*, Quilp threatens Kit's little brother that he will "make faces at [him] and throw [him] into fits" (*OCS*, 223). In *Martin Chuzzlewit*, young Martin – misinterpreting Tom Pinch's agitation – warns him that he shouldn't "drink too much of that sour wine, or you'll have a fit of some sort" (*MC*, 154). There are also "fits" which can be taken to mean paroxysms, as in *Dombey and Son:* "Captain Cuttle, in a fit of delirium" (*DS*, 730). A frequent use of "fits" is in the sense of hysterics, especially when used in connection with women. For example, in *Nicholas Nickleby*, Mr Lillyvick has decided to marry Miss Petowker and has kept his plans secret from the Kenwigs family:

> If my niece and the children had known a word about it before I came away, they'd have gone into fits at my feet, and never have come out of 'em till I took an oath not to marry anybody (*NN*, 322).

The term is, therefore, rather general and does not always bear only one meaning. Dickens uses the term as both other laymen and members of the medical profession have used it – and still use it.

Dickensian characters who clearly appear to be epileptic

Dickens's first description of epilepsy adheres to traditional beliefs and is used as the "outward and visible sign of [a total lack of] inward and spiritual grace" to borrow from the Anglican *Book of Common Prayer*. Edward Leeford, alias Monks, in *Oliver Twist*, is a villain and the fact that he is epileptic enforces the moral indignation the reader was to feel. The epileptologist, Professor Peter Wolf of the Mara Hospital in Bielefeld, Germany, writes:

> Monks is described as a ruthless half-criminal, governed by hatred and base inclination. The prejudice which relates epilepsy to criminality, which we still must fight today, seems to have existed already in Dickens' time.[14]

Despite some medical progress in terms of theory during the eighteenth century, there was still little help available for epileptics at the time *Oliver Twist* was written. The traditional view of a sort of demon possession still played a role in the public attitude towards the sufferer. It is interesting that although seizures were a defining characteristic of Monks, only one severe episode is actually described.[15]

Monks is intent on criminalizing his half-brother, Oliver, to rob him of his inheritance and to this end, the housebreaker, Bill Sikes, takes Oliver along to help commit a robbery. During the attempt, Oliver is shot and left for dead. By chance, Monks sees Oliver later and

> advanced towards Oliver, as if with the intention of aiming a blow at him, but fell violently on the ground: writhing and foaming, in a fit (*OT*, 217).

Oliver, not knowing who the man is, thinks Monks must be mad. There is possibly something of a *double entendre* here. On the one hand, Monks had muttered things which Oliver could not comprehend, and on the other, as noted above, epileptics were frequently put into the insane wards of workhouses or insane asylums.

A second episode is less dramatic. Monks arranges to meet Mr and Mrs Bumble to gain possession of the evidence of Oliver's identity. A flash of lightning and a peal of thunder elicit a seizure:

> He remained silent for a few moments; and then, removing his hands suddenly from his face, showed, . . .that it was much distorted and discoloured.

'These fits come over me, now and then,' said Monks, . . . ' and thunder sometimes brings them on' (*OT*, 251).

Later, Nancy describes Monks to Mr Brownlow:

His lips are often discoloured and disfigured with the marks of teeth; for he has desperate fits, and sometimes even bites his hands and covers them with wounds (*OT*, 314/5).

Monks is the only character in Dickens's works whom Professor Wolf regards as definitely epileptic. In personal correspondence, Professor Wolf expressed the opinion that

[i]t is rather safe to assume that Monk's seizures were understood by the author as epilepsy, even if he doesn't use the term. Everything else (in an article by Dr John Cosnett in *Epilepsia*) is questionable.[16]

Tissot considers sexual excess as one cause of epilepsy, stating that it has

been proven beyond doubt . . . that the strongest persons who had never previously suffered epilepsy have contracted the same through sexual excesses.

Those who indulge in sexual excess generally are victims of this disease, especially if they also consume excessive quantities of wine or other distilled beverages and brandies.[17]

Given the prevalence of sexually-transmitted diseases, especially various forms of syphilis, in the Victorian Age, it appears likely that Dickens was referring to syphilis when Mr Brownlow confronted Monks:

You . . . in whom all evil passions, vice and profligacy, festered, till they found a vent in a hideous disease which has made your face an index even to your mind . . . (*OT*, 336).

Professor Wolf had interpreted this as referring to the bite marks on Monks's lower lip in Nancy's description, but he accepted the possibility of my suggestion that perhaps Mr Brownlow meant syphilis. In light of Tissot's text, either would be plausible. It is also interesting to note that the first publication on epilepsy by the famous epileptologist, John Hughlings Jackson (1835-1911), nearly 30 years after publication of *Oliver Twist*, concerned "Cases of Epilepsy Associated with Syphilis."[18]

The second character suffering from epilepsy is the most detailed account of the three and is found in *Bleak House*. The law stationer, Snagsby, and his wife have a house-maid called Guster, who was hired cheap from the workhouse because, although she had been contracted, or farmed, during her growing time to an amiable benefactor of his species resident at Tooting and can not have failed to grow up under the most favourable of circumstances, has fits, which the parish can't account for (*BH*, 118).

Unlike Monks, Guster is not epileptic as a sign of her own evil, but of the evil of "baby farms" – a nineteenth-century institution for the "care" of orphans and pauper children. With the word "Tooting", Dickens made this clear to his contemporary readers – at least those in or near London. Guster is portrayed as one victim of Mr Bartholomew Drouet, master of a workhouse orphanage at Tooting. In 1849, 150 of the 1300 children at the institution died of cholera. This high number of deaths resulted in an obviously long-overdue inspection by the medical officers, who found that the cholera victims were placed 3-4 in one bed in a dank, ill-ventilated room above an open sewer, where they were left largely to their own devices and in their own filth. The children who did not have cholera were housed only marginally better; they were inadequately clothed, given food unfit for human consumption, and also physically abused. Dickens wrote four scathing articles in *The Examiner* at the time: "The Paradise at Tooting", "The Tooting Farm," "A Recorder's Charge" and "A Verdict for Mr Drouet". The latter article concerned the fact that Drouet, indicted for manslaughter in the case of one little boy who had died, was acquitted on the technicality that the child was already undernourished and would have died of cholera had he contracted the disease elsewhere.

In describing Guster, Dickens apparently was aware that epilepsy may result from cranial trauma in physical abuse. This is implicit in the young woman's association with Tooting at all, and especially in the report that

[Guster] is so apprehensive of being returned on the hands of her patron saint, that except when she is found with her head in the pail, or the sink, or the copper, or the dinner, or anything else that happens to be near her at the time of her seizure, she is always at work (*BH*, 119).

This association of epilepsy with cranial trauma in abuse is reported in Tissot's work:

Boretius (*de epilepsia ex depressione cranii*, 1725) reports on a young person who became epileptic because of harsh treatment by a schoolmaster, and in whom he held that the problem was caused by a depression of the cranium . . . [resulting] from the beatings he had received about the head.[19]

Considering cranial trauma as a possible cause of epilepsy, Tissot expresses an opinion which is in excellent accord with Dickens's own, on a matter close to Dickens's heart:

I have seen many children [between 4 and 12 years of age] who had become epileptic because of fright, *or abuse in schools by teachers, who were better qualified to be mule drivers than teachers.*[20]

It surprises somewhat that Dickens did not portray epileptic children at any of the three brutal schools in his novels. One might expect Squeers's (*NN*) or Creakle's (*DC*) treatment to result in seizures in at least some of the children. At the Charitable Grinders School in *Dombey and Son*, the children were

huffed and cuffed, and flogged and badged, and taught, as parrots are, by a brute jobbed into his place of schoolmaster with as much fitness for it as a hound (*DS*, 296).

It would not have been implausible to have epilepsy used as one sign of Rob the Grinder's "going wrong". It would undoubtedly, however, have limited his usefulness in other ways.

The description of Guster includes the fact that she was sometimes able to suppress the onset of seizures:

But downstairs is the charitable Guster, holding by the handrail of the kitchen stairs, and warding off a fit, as yet doubtfully, the same having been induced by Mrs Snagsby's screaming (*BH,* 332).

There are two possible origins of the fit, and they may both have been known to Dickens. The first and perhaps more likely is that Guster was frightened by Mrs Snagsby's screaming. It is, however, possible that the sound of the screams alone could provoke a seizure. Tissot reports that "a loud, unexpected and sharp-sounding noise often elicits such an effect" and it is recognized today that not only noises, but also colours, odours and certain movements may elicit seizures in persons disposed to such events.

Mr Snagsby, who is more sympathetic to Guster than his wife, realised both the relationship between the fright and seizures, and that Guster is able sometimes to suppress the onset. Snagsby tells the solicitor, Mr Tulkinghorn:

Now Guster . . . is timid and has fits, and she, taking fright at the foreigner's looks . . . gave way to it, instead of bearing up against it, and tumbled down the kitchen stairs out of one into another, such fits as I do sometimes think are never gone into, or come out of, in any house but ours (*BH*, 537).

This description would, according to the lecture by Dr Wilks cited above, have precluded that Guster is epileptic. Dr Wilks reported on "a patient with up to 12 'fits' a day. The frequency of the fits was also against the idea of genuine epilepsy, as real epileptic fits seldom recurred daily."[21] Modern medical science cedes the point in this case to Dickens and not to the physician writing nearly 20 years after publication of *Bleak House*. John Cosnett's article "Charles Dickens and Epilepsy"[22] interprets the description of Guster's seizures as *status epilepticus*. This could be questioned. To fit the definition, Guster must have lost consciousness at the beginning and not regained consciousness until the last seizure abated. Dickens describes "a chain of fits, with short intervals between" and says nothing of the state of consciousness. If Guster did not remain unconscious, the proper designation would be "serial seizures".

Even less clear is the interpretation of Guster's "staring and vacant" state while Mr Chadband is "preaching". Professor Wolf rejected the idea that Dickens may have been describing absence epilepsy, but Cosnett disagrees. He at least considers the possibility that "Guster was also subject to *petit mal*, accounting for such absence episodes."[23] Professor Wolf thought that Guster was just being "absent-minded," which would certainly be plausible; anyone not susceptible to the Chadband form of oratory would undoubtedly either leave the room or, if egress is prohibited, take refuge in just not listening. This may well have been the case with Guster, who would have evoked the wrath of Mrs Snagsby had she left the room. The state would appear to have lasted too long to depict classical absence epilepsy. There is, however, a possibility of *status petit mal*, in which attacks may last 30 minutes or up to 12 or more hours. The diagnosis could also be complex partial (temporal lobe) epilepsy, in which such attacks are possible.[24]

In writing about absence epilepsy, Dr John Hughlings Jackson used the term "dreamy states" and Dickens had some personal experience along those lines. His eldest son, Charlie, was to be sent to school, paid for by Angela Burdett-Coutts. In deciding where to send the boy, Dickens wrote to Miss Coutts on December 1, 1845:

> We have no reason to think that Charlie has anything but a vigorous constitution and good sound health. But when he is in full school employment, there is a strange kind of fading comes over him sometimes: the like of which, I don't think I ever saw.[25]

Since there is no other evidence, it would be inappropriate to take this as proof positive. It does, however, raise a slight suspicion that the boy may have suffered *petit mal* in childhood.

There is also other mention of epilepsy in the Dickens family, even in Dickens himself. All mention is, however, unsubstantiated and Professor Wolf warns that it is always safe to have some reserve when such a claim is made because this happens often, concerning whatever celebrity, and it is surely more common that the assumption is wrong than the opposite.[26]

The fact remains, however, that the claim that Dickens's sister, Laetitia, was "a delicate child, subject to fits" is made in *The Charles Dickens Encyclopedia.*"[27] That Dickens himself was epileptic in childhood is claimed in two books on epilepsy. Dr Matthew Woods makes the statement that

> Molière, Charles Dickens, Charles V, and Peter the Great also had fits, but only during childhood. Thus the reflex spasms of infancy may usually be prevented from developing into chronic epilepsy.[28]

Woods neither says *how* this prevention was effected, nor – even more importantly – does he cite his source.

The statement is quoted in the book by Lennox, mentioned above, citing only Woods as the source; Lennox's book, in turn, was used by an agency creating advertising for an antiepileptic product manufactured by a Canadian pharmaceutical company. A double full-page advertisement showed twelve historical "epileptics," including Dickens. Further "support" was found by the agency in a passage from Dr Hughlings Jackson's works. Hughlings Jackson wrote about a patient who reported a particular omen preceding his seizures, and referred to the following passage from *David Copperfield:*

> We have all some experience of a feeling which comes over us occasionally, of what we are saying and doing having been said or done before, in a remote time – of our having been surrounded, dim ages ago, by the same faces, objects and circumstances – of our knowing perfectly what will be said next, as if we suddenly remembered it.[29]

Apparently, since *David Copperfield* is known to be the most autobiographical of Dickens's novels, and this *déjà vu* experience was reported by David = Dickens, the advertising company drew the conclusion that David, hence Dickens, must have been epileptic. This is an extremely questionable conclusion, since most people have such experiences, but most people are not epileptic. At the Epilepsy Congress in Sydney, Australia in 1998, this advertisement was observed by a Dickensian, who submitted an incensed letter (unsigned) to the editor of *The Dickensian* at the very thought that Dickens might have been epileptic. Thus, we have confirmation of Professor Wolf's comments about the stigmatization still associated with epilepsy.

The final probably epileptic character is Walter Wilding, in the Christmas story written by Dickens and Wilkie Collins in 1867. Entitled "No Thoroughfare", the story is of a man who was adopted from the Hospital for Foundling Children. On his adopted mother's death, the man learns that he was adopted in place of another boy by mistake. This man of confused identity is given a form of epilepsy which is described as "being confused." The seizures are apparently heralded by "an old singing in [his] head." Toward the end of his life

> There began to creep over him a cloudy consciousness of often-recurring confusion in his head. He would unaccountably lose, sometimes whole hours, sometimes a whole day and night.[30]

He takes to his bed and says to his nurse/housekeeper: "I must of late have been subject to fits." Although "fits" is the word used to describe a variety of attack-like events, this character has been viewed in medical literature as definitely epileptic. The writer of Dickens's obituary in the *British Medical Journal* of June 18, 1870 stated that "His descriptions of epilepsy in Walter Wilding . . . show the hand of a master."[31] It could be asked here: which master? Wilkie Collins also wrote about epileptics, for example in "Poor Miss Finch" (1872), and Professor Wolf commented that

> Eliot and Collins shared that sense of professional quality characteristic of the great English realist authors of the last century.. . . One of the consequences is that their epileptic characters are depicted according to the best available medical information . . . with sympathy and dignity.[32]

Characters suffering isolated seizures

There are two characters in Dickens's novels in this category. The first is Anthony Chuzzlewit in *Martin Chuzzlewit*. Anthony is discussed in detail in the chapter on stroke, but he is mentioned here, since an epileptiform seizure preceded his stroke. The knowledge that seizures may be associated with stroke is not common among laymen. This is an instance in which Dickens's writing is surprisingly accurate – and for which his source remains unknown. It is noted that the surgeon bled the patient and that "some remedies" were applied. Since the novel was written before the use of bromides (first used by Charles Locock in 1857), it is a question of what might have been applied. According to Tissot, it was useless to use smelling salts, but the use of camphor, quinine, or mistletoe, among other phytotherapeutics, was common.

The second character is in the last of Dickens's completed novels, *Our Mutual Friend* (1863-65). The schoolteacher, Bradley Headstone, is a very repressed individual, who subjects himself to extremely rigid self-discipline. He falls in love with his pupil's sister, Lizzie Hexam, who is pursued by Eugene Wrayburn. Jealous, believing that Lizzie loves Eugene, Headstone attacks him and throws him, nearly dead, into the river. Lizzie saves him – demonstrating that Dickens was aware of the effect of adrenaline, even if he probably did not understand the mechanism enabling a young woman to carry her injured lover from a boat to an inn on the shore, though she would normally not be able to even lift the weight.

Later, when Headstone learns that, not only was his murder attempt unsuccessful, but Lizzie and Eugene are to be married,

> He was took very bad to be sure, and was biting and knocking about (the man said) furiously (*OMF*, 821).

Headstone remembers this incident as

> Fate . . . having put a fraud upon him – overreached him – and in his impotent mad rage bit, and tore, and had his fit (*OMF*, 863).

Headstone, whose conscience has been tormenting him – not with what he had done, but how he should have done it better – is close to total nervous collapse.

> This horrible condition brought on other fits. He could not have said how many, or when, but he saw in the faces of his pupils that they had seen him in that state, and that they were possessed by a dread of his relapsing (*OMF*, 864).

Roger (Rogue) Riderhood, whom Headstone had tried to implicate in the crime by copying his attire, threatens blackmail. Riderhood turns up unexpectedly while Headstone is teaching and nearly causes an immediate seizure:

> [Headstone] sat down on a stool which one of his boys had put for him, and he had a passing knowledge that he was in danger of falling, and that his face was becoming distorted. But, the fit went off for that time, and he wiped his mouth, and stood up again (*OMF,* 864).

After Riderhood tells Headstone that he found the clothes he wore and knows that he committed the attempted murder, he

> slouched out of the school, leaving the master to get through his weary work as he might, and leaving the whispering pupils to observe the master's face until he fell into the fit which had been long impending (*OMF*, 867).

Remembering Tissot's statement that violent emotions may result in epilepsy, it would appear that Dickens had epileptiform seizures in mind in describing Bradley Headstone. But Professor Wolf disagrees. In his words:

> The schoolroom scene is a psychodynamic reaction *in extremis,* of a physically exhausted, emotionally deeply disturbed person who finds himself caught in a fix of

which he sees no way out. Of course he's in a "state" but nothing indicates an epileptic seizure.[33]

From a lay-literary point of view, however, it is plausible that Bradley Headstone is a "respectable" version of Monks. There are, after all, no "fits" described until he has committed a crime, and what was for him likely even worse, lost control of himself. This would appear to have given rise to the same symptoms as resulted from Monks's profligacy, even though it would undoubtedly be incorrect to say that Headstone was epileptic.

The final figure to be considered is John Jasper in the unfinished *The Mystery of Edwin Drood.* There is only one brief mention, when Drood says of his uncle, Jasper:

> What I mean is, that he is subject to a kind of paroxysm, or fit – I saw him in it once – and I don't know but that so great a surprise coming upon him direct from me whom he is so wrapped up in, might bring it on perhaps (*ED*, 118).

Looking back across Dickens's descriptions of epileptics/epileptiform seizures, it would appear that, in this respect, Jasper may be a composite of Monks's evil and Headstone's loss of control, as well as a reflection of Guster in Drood's recognition of surprise as a factor eliciting seizures. The "family resemblance" between Jasper and Headstone is also noted by W. Robson, particularly in the scene in which Jasper declares his passion for Rosa. Robson thinks this may be "an artistic mistake, unless Felix Aylmer is right in thinking that it is a deliberate parody of Headstone."[34] We know nothing of the circumstances of the fit but its probable interpretation as a force beyond Jasper's control and outward sign of malignancy of character. The *medical* question, which must remain unanswered, can be raised here whether Jasper, an opium addict, had suffered withdrawal symptoms, expressed as an epileptiform seizure, in Drood's presence. That Dickens was aware of this possibility is not unlikely, given the widespread use of various forms of opium in the nineteenth century (see Chapter 7), the dawning awareness of the habituation potential of the drug, DeQuincey's descriptions of withdrawal problems, and Dickens's friendship with Wilkie Collins, who was addicted due to treatment for chronic pain.

Conclusion

As with other morbid states, Dickens wrote with considerable accuracy about epilepsy or epileptiform seizures. The assumption is plausible that Dickens was aware of what was being published in medical journals and it is beyond doubt that he observed people suffering seizures. The connection between epileptiform seizure and stroke in the elderly is not commonly known among laymen and the description of Anthony Chuzzlewit must contribute to our admiration of Dickens as a narrator of medical realism. The connection leads now into a chapter on stroke, which is the most common medicopathological state after tuberculosis in Dickens's works.

---

[1] S. Ried, G. Schűler (1994), 5 [my translation].
[2] Hippocrates (Adam translation 1849) II, 843; quoted in: Lennox (1960) I, 13.
[3] Temkin (1971), 285.
[4] Temkin (1971), 263.
[5] Lecture by Dr Gabriel Andral (1797-1876), Professor of Pathology and Therapy, *The Lancet* 1832-33: 64-71 and 102-105.
[6] From Wolf (1994), 6.
[7] Tissot (1771), 39 [All quotes from Tissot are my translation from a German edition of 1771.]
[8] Temkin (1971), 263.
[9] *Edinburgh Medical Journal* 21, 1824:204.
[10] Temkin (1971), 257.
[11] *On-line Medical Dictionary, University of Newcastle upon Tyne, 1997-2003 (Oct 6, 1997).*
[12] Temkin (1971), 258.
[13] *The Lancet*, Nov. 28, 1998, 1750.
[14] Wolf (1995), S12.
[15] A recent BBC production has Monks suffering a seizure practically every time he appears on screen.
[16] Personal communication dated March 26, 1998.
[17] Tissot (1771), 61, 62.
[18] Published in the *Medical Times and Gazette* 1 1861: 648-52; 2:59-60.
[19] Tissot (1771), 90.
[20] Tissot (1771), 186, my emphasis.
[21] Wilks, *The Lancet*, February 26, 1870.
[22] Cosnett (1994). This was the article referred to by Prof. Wolf, see above.
[23] Ibid, 904.
[24] Browne and Feldman: *Epilepsy: diagnosis and management.* Cited by Dr Cosnett, personal communication, December 13, 2001.
[25] *Letters* 4. 442.
[26] Personal communication, March 26, 1998.
[27] Michael and Mollie Hardwick (1973), 342. No source is given for the information.
[28] Woods (1913), 293.
[29] This is the version cited by Hughlings Jackson; the Clarendon text is shorter [*DC,* 311].
[30] Ticknor and Fields, Boston edition of 1867, 18.
[31] *BMJ,* June 18,1870, 636.
[32] Wolf (1995), S14.
[33] Personal communication, April 2, 1998.
[34] Robson, 142, citing Aylmer "The Drood Case" (1964).

CHAPTER 4: Stroke

This chapter addresses what appears to be stroke. This is the second most common pathological construct in Dickens's works after tuberculosis. No fewer than eleven (possibly twelve) characters suffer some form of this disorder, in novels from *Pickwick Papers* to *Great Expectations*. As usual with Dickens, the circumstances are individualized and, while medically plausible, are tailored to suit the novel with respect to cause, timing, circumstances and outcome. Various symptom clusters are depicted, so that the interested clinician might be enabled, in light of today's knowledge, to define the affected areas of the brain.

An article published in 1829 will serve to review what was known of stroke at the time. It was defined as

> a pathological state of the brain, characterized by the sudden suppression of higher nerve functions, consciousness, the senses and voluntary motions, in which however the lower or so-called vital functions, especially respiration and blood circulation, continue largely unimpaired.[1]

My discussion centres on the descriptions of stroke in the novels and a possible interpretation – in this case literary as well as medical – of Dickens's use of the disorder. Where possible, comments by medical writers are given, but, remarkably enough, many of these characters elicited no comment in medical or hospital journals, despite being characters of some importance to the novel. The literary use is examined because it has revealed a not hitherto-identified predisposing factor in characters afflicted with stroke.

Rather than being discussed in chronological order of creation, the characters are grouped according to various criteria, starting with those in whom stroke is immediately fatal, followed by stroke resulting from violent emotion. A third section discusses stroke as a clearly literary device. Stroke as retribution for emotional and religious rigidity is observed in more than one character and one final victim is postulated about whom there is disagreement between literary and medical interpretation. The discussion closes with the strokes of Mrs Skewton and Sir Leicester Dedlock, which Dickens described in considerable detail.

Dickens's descriptions of immediately-fatal stroke

Consistent with reality, several of Dickens's stroke victims die immediately. The first such character is in one of the interpolated stories in *Pickwick Papers*: "The Convict's Return" in Chapter 6. A young man, who had been transported for theft, returns to the village where he had grown up. Meanwhile his mother has died and he encounters only his father – a workhouse inmate who had abused him and his mother. The old man becomes terrified at seeing his son and strikes the young man; the young man begins to defend himself, then lets his arms drop by his side.

> The old man uttered a loud yell ... His face turned black: the gore rushed from his mouth and nose, and dyed the grass a deep dark red, as he staggered and fell. He had ruptured a blood-vessel: and he was a dead man before his son could raise him from that thick, sluggish pool (*PP*, 74).

This gory end is a "sensational journalist's" description of apoplexy elicited by emotional stress, which is the causative agent in several of Dickens's portrayals of stroke. The brutality of the man's treatment of his wife and son is punished by violent death but not at the hands of the person brutalized. '"Vengeance is mine; . . ." saith the Lord'[2] undoubtedly came immediately to mind among Dickens's Bible-literate contemporaries.

Three later figures can be identified and quickly dealt with, since only one of these strokes occurred during the course of the narrative, and none was described in any detail. The earliest of these is Francis Spenlow in *David Copperfield.* Death occurs offstage and as a device to remove an obstacle to the hero's achieving his desires. Spenlow, who knew that his daughter Dora was not provided for, would never have allowed her to marry a penniless suitor, so he had to be done away with to suit the plot.[3] The death is described as follows:

> Whether [Mr Spenlow] fell out [of his carriage] in a fit, or got out, feeling ill before the fit came on - or even whether he was dead then, though there is no doubt he was quite insensible - no one appears to know. If he breathed, certainly he never spoke. Medical assistance was got as soon as possible, but it was quite useless (*DC*, 454).

Here Dickens uses the term "fit". As discussed in connection with epilepsy, the term can be seen in Dickens's works to denote practically everything from voluntary, theatrical female manipulative hysterics (as with Mrs Varden and Miggs in *BR*) to epilepsy or epileptiform convulsions (like Monks in *OT*) to apoplexy or stroke, as in this case. Its connotation here for Dickens would appear to be mainly loss of control and/or of dignity. My assumption in the case of Spenlow is that "fit" is used to refer to stroke and indicates loss of Spenlow's control over Dora. It may be, of course, that epileptiform convulsions are also implied. Possibly Dickens correlated this with the case of Anthony Chuzzlewit, since the illustration of Chuzzlewit in his seizure, discussed below, bears the legend "The Dissolution of Partnership" and Chapter 38 in *Copperfield* is headed with nearly the identical words: "A Dissolution of Partnership."

The second such death is that of Josiah Bounderby in *Hard Times* (1854):

> Had he any prescience of the day, five years to come, when Josiah Bounderby of Coketown was to die of a fit in the Coketown street (*HT,* 312).

The most likely diagnosis in the case of Bounderby would appear to be apoplexy. Bounderby is a choleric, explosive type, who is very jealous of his bogus "self-made-man" status. It is therefore poetic justice that lets Dickens conceive an undignified public death for a man whose false pride and blustering manner isolate him from the society he wishes to dominate.

A parallel case to Bounderby is Joe Gargery's father in *Great Expectations*, who has died before the novel begins. Not only was the elder Mr Gargery reportedly choleric, but also an alcoholic, abusive husband and father. Joe's description of his father's death is not clear as to the actual cause. In his characteristic language, Joe says his father "went off in a purple leptic fit." This could be a transcription of either "apoplectic" or "epileptic" and either could result from alcohol abuse. The more likely interpretation would tend toward apoplectic because Gargery appears to be the same sort of character as the convict's father. The stroke in both cases was apparently sudden, violent and immediately fatal.

Cerebral insults precipitated by violent emotion

As mentioned above, violent emotion is posited as the cause of cerebral insult in many, but not all, of Dickens's stroke victims. The earliest stroke victim actually belonging to the novel in which he appears is John Willet (*BR*, 1841). While the Maypole is ransacked, Willet loses his senses, not really comprehending what has befallen him:

> John Willet, left alone in his dismantled bar, continued to sit staring about him; awake as to his eyes, certainly, but with all his powers of reason and reflection in a sound and dreamless sleep (*BR*, 500).

This shock is one from which Willet never recovers; he "remained in the same mental condition down to the last moment of his life" (*BR,* 736). Whether there is, in fact, a slight cerebral insult involved at this stage is unclear, though I have assumed so for the purposes of grouping. Later, Willet is attacked – for unknown reasons - with

> the symptoms of apoplexy. . . . [T]he doctors all agreed . . . that he ought to die, and took it very ill that he did not, he remained alive - possibly on account of his constitutional slowness - for nearly seven years more, when he was one morning found speechless in his bed (*BR*, 736).

He regains consciousness one week later and then dies.

Current knowledge recognizes a non-vascular process in this slow downhill course. If much had not been made earlier of Willet's slowness, a concurrent *abulia* (syndrome of slowness, lack of spontaneity, and laconic spoken or motor responses of various etiologies) could be postulated, but if it is present, it predates the ransacking of the Maypole. The readers' introduction to Willet is to a man whose boast was that

> if he were slow, he was sure; which assertion could in one sense at least, be by no means gainsaid, seeing that he was in everything unquestionably the reverse of fast . . . (*BR*, 45).

Interpretations of John Willet and the Maypole range from John Forster's statement that "John Willet is a genuinely comic creation"[4] to Gordon Spence's "part of the humorous and grotesque characterization that the presentation of Mr Bumble . . . has led us to expect."[5] But there is a darker side to Willet's nature and, I think, to his symbolic role, of which his stroke appears to be part. Willet tyrannizes his son Joe, unable to accept any form of change, including the fact that Joe is no longer a child. He may be a grotesque representation of the exaggerated paternalism of English society at that time. The fate which Willet suffers, Dickens seems to be saying, is that which will surely befall the country if the conditions conducive to unleashing mob violence are not dealt with. In Spence's view, Dickens makes "the burning of Newgate symbolic of a general revolt of chaotic and irrational impulses against an oppressive authority."[6] Pointing out the various father/son conflicts which run through the novel, Spence would apparently see the *Leitmotiv* typical of much of Dickens's writing: "Barnaby and Hugh, who become leaders of the mob, are, respectively, idiotic and bestial owing to the criminality and irresponsibility of their unknown fathers."[7] This may be slightly unfair to Barnaby, who, rather than being "idiotic", has been viewed as autistic,[8] whose father was not unknown in the sense of illegitimacy like Hugh's and who can hardly be said to be a "leader of the mob."

The case is different with John Willet, who is not unknown to his son; he faces his responsibility as a parent to the extent which his limited intellect permits, but his inflexibility leads inevitably to rebellion in his son and, while not resulting in criminal behaviour, does result indirectly in mutilation. Willet's cerebral insult finalizes the rigidity of his thought processes and curtails physical movement, thus creating a space in which the younger generation can finally act.

A similar episode is postulated in *David Copperfield* (1849-50) in the figure of Mrs Steerforth. As in the case of Willet - assuming a slight stroke as a result of the pillaging of the Maypole - her stroke is precipitated by violent emotional shock. After the storm in Yarmouth, David Copperfield takes it on himself to escort Steerforth's body home and break the news to his mother:

Mrs Steerforth, fallen back stiffly in her chair, and making no sound but a moan, cast her eyes upon [Rosa] with a wide stare (*DC*, 653).

The moan the mother uttered, from time to time, went to my heart. Always the same. Always inarticulate and stifled. . . . Always proceeding from a rigid mouth and closed teeth, as if the jaw were locked and the face frozen up in pain (*DC*, 653).

Later in the day, I returned, and we laid him in his mother's room. She was just the same, they told me; Miss Dartle never left her; doctors were in attendance, many things had been tried; but she lay like a statue, except for the low sound now and then (*DC*, 655).

The first of these quotations is strongly reminiscent of John Willet in his demolished bar. There is the vacant, uncomprehending stare and lack of articulation. It could, perhaps, be argued that Mrs Steerforth has lost her reason - a not impossible interpretation considering her total fixation on her son. The case can be pressed just as strongly, however, for a cerebral insult as the basis for the rigidity and lack of articulation, especially considering the description of the "face frozen up in pain," which could be indicative of the contorted facial features commonly observed in stroke victims.

Most conspicuous, however is the phrase "she lay like a statue" in the third passage quoted. Like Willet a "single parent," Mrs Steerforth goes to the opposite extreme and is overindulgent of her son. In her own way, however, she is as inflexible and tyrannical as old John Willet. Mrs Steerforth and James are both obstinate and wilful, vying against each other for control. While he lies dead in her house, she becomes physically immoveable and appears in some measure to share his fate in retribution for her rigidity and lack of positive control over her son's moral formation. Mrs Steerforth's rigidity in dealing with James at the end of his life becomes corporealised in her lying "like a statue" without the power to change her ways or make amends. She recovers to a limited extent, reportedly with a "countenance in which there are some traces of old pride and beauty, feebly contending with a querulous, imbecile, fretful, wandering of the mind" (*DC*, 715). The querulousness, fretfulness and wandering of the mind are typical sequelae of certain forms of stroke and again show Dickens's grasp of the disorder and its results.

Stroke as a literary device

While the cases discussed thus far all have a purpose within the novel, stroke appears to have been used – with the exception of Francis Spenlow – as an observed medical plausibility under the circumstances described. In contrast to this, *Martin Chuzzlewit* includes stroke as a literary device selected for its dramatic presentation. In Anthony Chuzzlewit's case, the onset is sudden, unexpected, not associated with any violent emotion and accompanied by dramatic epileptiform convulsions. Clinically, the picture would likely be cerebral ischemia. The sounds Chuzzlewit makes when he is stricken are misinterpreted by Mr Pecksniff and Chuzzlewit's son, Jonas, who, looking around

> saw Anthony Chuzzlewit extended on the floor, with the old clerk upon his knees beside him. He had fallen from his chair in a fit, and lay there, battling for each gasp of breath, . . . A young man in the fulness of his vigour, struggling with so much strength of desperation, would have been a dismal sight; but an old, old, shrunken body, endowed with preternatural might, and giving the lie in every motion of its every limb and joint to its enfeebled aspect, was a hideous spectacle indeed (*MC*, 306).

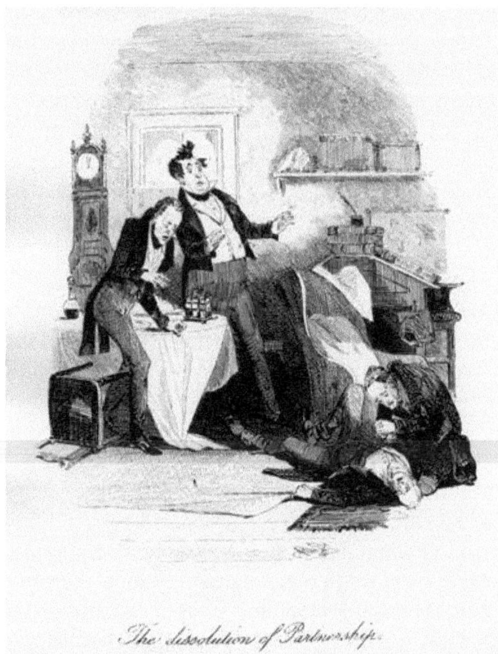

Fig. 5: "The Dissolution of Partnership". *Martin Chuzzlewit*. The Dickens Museum.

The day after the episode, Anthony Chuzzlewit appears, dressed, in the room where his son and Pecksniff are sitting. He is very near death and - typical of certain forms of stroke - unable to articulate, though most certainly clear in his own mind what he was "saying":

> He spoke to them in something of his own voice . . . What he would have said, God knows. He seemed to utter words, but they were such as man had never heard.

And this was the most fearful circumstance of all, to see him standing there, babbling in an unearthly tongue (*MC*, 310).

The purpose for the plot here would clearly seem to be to unnerve Jonas Chuzzlewit. He believes that he has poisoned his father and is relieved that Pecksniff is in the house as his witness that he had given his father nothing prior to the attack. When, however, the stroke is not immediately fatal and Anthony Chuzzlewit appears, babbling, on the scene, Jonas's nervous tension is augmented, setting in train the subsequent events. Dickens gives no clue that Chuzzlewit was being accusatory, and later the old clerk, Chuffy, relates that Chuzzlewit had found the poison and not taken any, though pretending to do so. He had taken on himself the blame for the attempted murder, recognizing it as the result of training his son to be greedy and selfish. This is perhaps what he was trying to say, but couldn't articulate, shortly before he died. For Jonas Chuzzlewit, the interpretation is accusatory in response to his own guilty conscience.

Stroke and religious/moral rigidity

Unchristian behaviour in characters who are loudest in professing their religion is the butt of Dickens's satire in several cases – Mr Stiggins (*PP*) and Mr Chadband (*BH*) come to mind. But worse than such, for Dickens, are those whose religion is based on Old Testament harshness and repression. Dickens's use of stroke to express the moral rigidity of such characters is exemplified first by Miss Barbary in *Bleak House*. Stern and unforgiving to her natural niece, Esther, with neither affection nor encouragement but only blame and wrath for the puzzled and timid child, Miss Barbary is struck down and neither moves nor speaks for the seven days until her death. It is as if the illness is a metaphor for divine vengeance – appropriately, since Miss Barbary is a great believer in the kind of Old Testament God Dickens abhorred.

One stroke victim in *Little Dorrit* (1855-57) is a psychological study of its own for most of the book and further exemplifies Dickens's metaphoric use of stroke. Carrying through the dominant theme of various forms of imprisonment, Dickens created Mrs Clennam. Bound by her own will to a wheelchair, her environment limited to one dull room in a decaying house, Mrs Clennam seeks to justify in terms of rigid, uncharitable, unforgiving Protestant fundamentalism her behaviour toward Arthur's father and Arthur, who believes he is her son but is really his father's illegitimate son by another woman. An even more clearly delineated figure than Miss Barbary, Dickens uses Mrs Clennam to attack those who would make Sunday a bleak day of strict discipline,[9] and especially those who would abuse the Bible by interpreting it for their own purposes.

Left ambiguous to the end of the novel, the self-imposed nature of Mrs Clennam's imprisonment is emphasised by her rising from her chair, leaving her house and rushing to the Marshalsea to prevent Arthur's learning the truth of his birth. Rigaud, the blackmailer, waits in the house and - as Mrs Clennam returns there - the rotten beams finally give way, the house collapses, burying Rigaud and his evil, and explaining by-the-bye the sounds which had frightened the serving woman, Affery.[10]

In parallel to the collapse of the building is the collapse of "The House" - if one takes Mrs Clennam to be the sole surviving member of the business. For, as the house collapsed, she suffered a stroke:

> There, Mrs Clennam dropped upon the stones; and she never from that hour moved so much as a finger again, or had the power to speak one word. For upwards of three years ... she lived and died a statue (*LD*, 772).

The theme of Old Testament religious fundamentalism is again portrayed in a surrogate mother figure, as it was in Miss Barbary. Rigidity of heart and mind is punished with rigidity of body in divine retribution.

Like Mrs Steerforth, Miss Barbary and Mrs Clennam had done violence to human feelings and human relationships. For Dickens, stroke, the severance of contact with the world around one, is the death such characters must die; internal rather than external violence, in the isolation of seeing without capacity to act, a "statue" – an immobile shell of self.

Stroke or uremia?

The one character for whom I postulate stroke for literary reasons, but for whom uremia is considered more likely in medical opinion, is found in *Little Dorrit.* William and Amy Dorrit are one of several inversions of the parent-child relationship in Dickens's works. Amy, the youngest of three children, is the only family member who is emotionally mature. She is the family's anchor, both emotionally and financially, while the father concerns himself with his supposed dignity of place as "Father of the Marshalsea", where he is incarcerated for the first part of the novel. After being released on inheriting great wealth, he and his family travel extensively and live abroad. Returned to Rome from London, having invested all his money with the swindler, Merdle, some changes are noted in his looks and behaviour. His mind begins to wander and he looks at Amy and around him as if he "needed assurance from his sense of sight that they were not in the old prison-room" (*LD*, 621).

He claims the following morning to have rested well, but he falls asleep several times and "[h]is fits of dozing were as sudden as they had been overnight, and were as short and profound" (*LD*, 623).

The use of "fits" is noted here. Thus far, nothing definitely pathological has been described; the term here simply signifies intermittent occurrence. An older man, just returned from an arduous journey under the conditions prevailing in the nineteenth century certainly has just cause to be tired, and fatigue alone could result in disorientation. But "fits", as noted earlier, often point to a loss of control and a loss of dignity; Dorrit was particularly jealous of his dignity. Clearly, Dickens is preparing the reader for Dorrit's final indignity.

The following day, Dorrit looks "indefinably shrunken and old". His breakdown is complete at Mrs Merdle's dinner party, where he suddenly becomes totally disoriented and believes himself in the Marshalsea. He is taken home, put to bed and dies ten days later. Monroe Engel – a medical layman novelist – cites the scene and says "... and when [Dorrit] suffers the stroke that precedes his death ..."[11] Apparently Engel considers the episode, as I do, from the significance stroke seems to have had for Dickens, that is the loss of dignity. Dorrit's dignity has been exposed for the sham it is fortunately for him, he is unaware of it.

According to Dr John Cosnett, the medical pattern here could be uremia or senile dementia,[12] except that the final phase was of more rapid onset and terminal within two weeks from the first mention of Dorrit's altered looks and behaviour. No paralysis is mentioned and there is no return to consciousness of reality, though a semblance of consciousness is reported: Dorrit sends Amy out to pawn possessions and remains, to the last, convinced that he is still in the Marshalsea, having no remembrance of the interval since his release.

In dying, Dorrit resembles John Willet, whose disorder was also in some measure indirectly elicited by being imprisoned - in Willet's case, being bound to a chair. With the scene at Mrs Merdle's dinner party, Dickens makes it clear to the reader that Dorrit's mind, kept under such strict governance since his physical release from prison, had, in fact, never left the prison at all. The tenor of the novel is that each person actually creates his or her own prison, even if this can be for a time more-or-less successfully concealed from the world outside - and indeed from oneself. The loss of control over the mind, the attendant loss of "dignity" occasioned by a cerebral *insult* – particularly fitting for William Dorrit! - reveals the existence of the inner prison and throws open the "cell" to the release found ultimately in death.

Two Dickensian "case reports"

Dickens presents the final two stroke victims in considerable detail. These provide excellent examples of his power of clinical observation and I shall therefore quote excerpts at more length than might otherwise be appropriate.

Mrs Skewton

We have seen the ways in which Dickens uses stroke to imply retribution, or to remove a hero's obstacle, or to deflate self-importance. How glaringly stroke can illustrate ludicrous, vain behaviour is seen in Mrs Skewton in *Dombey and Son.* Lord Brain, commenting in 1955 in "Dickensian Diagnoses," points out that Dickens's account of [Mrs Skewton's] illness is

> remarkable not only for the accuracy of his description of individual symptoms but even more, perhaps, for the skill with which he conveys the relentless progress of the disease, with its insidious onset and catastrophic exacerbations.[13]

Dickens gave this figure a great deal of attention while plotting and writing the novel and the description is both fascinating and horrifying. For anyone who has cared for a stroke victim, the realism is extremely moving.

This figure gives us one of the rare instances in which the *Working Notes* provide insight into motivation in relation to illness. The timetable for the novel uses Mrs Skewton's paralysis as a marker, with the first attack within six months after Edith's wedding to Dombey, then

> departure to Brighton for Mrs Skewton's health - the lapse of time at Brighton - and the period of Mrs Skewton's death, and the period after Mrs Skewton's death - say all in a space of One Year. . . . And a year is said to have taken place between Uncle Sol's disappearance and Mrs Skewton's first attack of Paralysis, which seems to agree, perfectly, with this calculation.

The paralysis was, then, an important event in the novel. But, as yet, there is no mention of the motivation behind it. Why should Mrs Skewton suffer a stroke? The Note for Chapter 36[14] "More Warnings Than One" reads:

> Death's warning to Mrs Skewton - Her paralysis - The change it makes in her.

Here we can begin to see - even without reading the novel - that Mrs Skewton is not just a secondary character who, in principle, need not have appeared at all.

Mrs Skewton is depicted from the first as a vain, ridiculous old woman, and it is mentioned later that she has palsy. The word is apparently used only in the sense of tremors, though the medical definition is actually paralysis. It would seem, however, that when Dickens wrote "paralysis," he was referring to the stroke itself.

Mrs Skewton denies encroaching age and physical weakness:

> I think I am a little nervous this morning, Flowers, . . . My hand quite shakes (*DS*, 552).

Shortly after a painful interview between Edith and Carker, Mrs Skewton has her first stroke. The trigger was not, however, violent emotion as in the cases discussed earlier, for:

> Mrs Skewton, reposing on her sofa, and sipping her chocolate, had heard nothing but the low word business, for which she had a mortal aversion. . . . Therefore Mrs Skewton asked no questions, and showed no curiosity (*DS*, 558).

She was being dressed for dinner when she was stricken. The maid, Flowers, reports her illness and that "she's making faces."

> They took her to pieces in very shame, and put the little of her that was real on a bed. Doctors were sent for, and soon came. Powerful remedies were resorted to; opinions given that she would rally from this shock, but would not survive another; and there she lay speechless, and staring at the ceiling, for days: sometimes making inarticulate sounds in answer to such questions as did she know who were present, and the like: sometimes giving no reply either by sign or gesture, or in her unwinking eyes.
>
> At length she began to recover consciousness, and in some degree the power of motion, though not yet of speech. One day the use of her right hand returned and showing it to her maid who was in attendance on her, and appearing very uneasy in her mind, she made signs for a pencil and some paper. This the maid immediately provided, thinking she was going to make a will, or write some last request; and Mrs Dombey being from home, the maid awaited the result with solemn feelings (*DS*, 559).

This is remarkably accurate as a brief description of a patient recovering from a stroke, with right hemiplegia and dysphasia. To this point, we can feel some pity for the woman, knowing that all her pretences have been torn to shreds. The narrator knows this; the reader knows this; the only one who doesn't - or refuses to - know this is Mrs Skewton herself. The text continues:

> After much painful scrawling and erasing, and putting in of wrong characters, which seemed to tumble out of the pencil of their own accord, the old woman produced this document:
>
> 'Rose-coloured curtains.'

The maid being perfectly transfixed, and with tolerable reason, Cleopatra amended the manuscript by adding two words more, when it stood thus:

'Rose-coloured curtains for doctors.'

The maid now perceived remotely that she wished these articles to be provided for the better presentation of her complexion to the faculty; . . . the rose-coloured curtains were added to her bed, and she mended with increased rapidity from that hour (*DS*, 559).

A typical Dickensian animation is noted in the characters "which ... tumble out of the pencil of their own accord." Lord Brain, commenting on this dysgraphia, reminds us of Dr Johnson on the effect of his stroke: "My hand, I knew not how nor why, made wrong letters."[15] The physical debility attending stroke, accurately depicted as it had been in two previous novels and would be again in three more, awakens first some feeling of pity, which Dickens turns on itself to disgust, showing that even debility and a near encounter with death have no power to change this woman from the vain, shallow creature she was prior to the attack. And Dickens isn't through with her yet. He goes on to show the changes which the stroke effects in her mind:

It was a tremendous sight to see this old woman in her finery leering and mincing at Death, and playing off her youthful tricks upon him as if he had been the Major; but an alteration in her mind that ensued on the paralytic stroke was fraught with as much matter for reflection, and was quite as ghastly (*DS*, 559).

In this one instance, Dickens identifies the "paralytic stroke" rather than describing a nameless disorder. The "playful" Mrs Skewton, who refused to take anything seriously - except herself - is turned by the stroke into a querulous, whining, demanding creature. Once again, Dickens uses realistic medical description to achieve his purpose. One of the most common effects of stroke on the personality is a tendency to cry - with or without an objectifiable reason: "[Mrs Skewton] would look at [Edith] . . . now with capricious tears and jealous shakings of the head" (*DS*, 604). The patient frequently becomes demanding: "hugely exacting in respect of Edith's affection and gratitude and attention to her" (*DS*, 560), and self-pity is a normal reaction to the physical debility: "let *me* rest in my out-of-the-way room, with no society and no attention" (*DS*, 561).

The inexorable approach of death following the stroke is the undercurrent of the remainder of this and the following chapter. Mrs Skewton recovers at least partially from the first stroke, dresses even more inappropriately for her age, and continues her denial pattern. An indistinctness of speech and an intermittent forgetfulness remain. On medical advice, Mrs Skewton is taken to Brighton:

Without having undergone any decided second attack of her malady, the old woman seemed to have crawled backward in her recovery from the first. She was more lean and shrunken, more uncertain in her imbecility, and made stranger confusions in her mind and memory (*DS*, 602).

The Note for Chapter 41 "New Voices in the Waves" tells us what Dickens has been leading up to:

> Mrs Skewton's death, in contrast with Paul's.

In reading the novel, many contrasts stand out, such as the two Carker brothers, Mr Dombey and Uncle Sol as businessmen, Florence and the children she sees in the house across the street, among many others. The reader has also noticed that there are two mother/daughter pairs and might expect that this contrast is the main one in which Mrs Skewton is involved. But the Notes cited above make it clear that Mrs Skewton's illness and death are, for Dickens, just as important as her life - if not actually more so. Apart from the fact that Dickens uses a revolutionary approach in describing Paul's illness only from the child's perspective, the contrast between the child's patient suffering, then his acceptance and embracing of death and the vain old woman's denial of even the normal aging process is powerfully presented.

Sir Leicester Dedlock

Several years after *Dombey and Son*, Dickens created one stroke victim who survives sentient and reasonably functional for an undefined period of years after the insult. This is Sir Leicester Dedlock in *Bleak House*, in whom Dickens described the phases of the disease in considerable and meticulous detail. As with John Willet and Mrs Steerforth, the attack is triggered by violent emotion - something with which the reader has been led to believe Sir Leicester had no experience. His solicitor, Tulkinghorn, having been murdered, Sir Leicester offers a reward for the capture of the murderer, only to learn from the detective, Mr Bucket, that Lady Dedlock is implicated in the crime. When he is first confronted with this fact, Sir Leicester is depicted as being afflicted with the onset of stroke:

> Something frozen and fixed is upon his manner, over and above its usual shell of haughtiness; and Mr Bucket soon detects an unusual slowness in his speech, and now and then a curious trouble in beginning, which occasions him to utter inarticulate sounds (*BH*, 669).

Later, when Bucket has arrested Lady Dedlock's former maid, Hortense, and left, Sir Leicester is stricken:

> At length he gazes round the empty room, and finding it deserted, rises unsteadily to his feet, pushes back his chair, and walks a few steps, supporting himself by the table. Then he stops; and with more of those inarticulate sounds, lifts up his

eyes and seems to stare at something. . . . And, even to the point of his sinking on the ground, oblivious of his suffering, he can yet pronounce her name with something like distinctness in the midst of those intrusive sounds (*BH*, 683/4).

Sir Leicester is not found for an unspecified number of hours, and he remains insensible to the end of the day:

. . . the day has ebbed away, and it is night in his room, before his stertorous breathing lulls, or his fixed eyes show any consciousness of the candle that is occasionally passed before them. But when this change begins, it goes on; and by-and-bye he nods, or moves his eyes, or even his hand, in token that he hears and comprehends.

He fell down, this morning, a handsome stately gentleman; somewhat infirm, but of a fine presence, and with a well-filled face. He lies upon his bed, an aged man with sunken cheeks, the decrepit shadow of himself. His voice was rich and mellow; and he had so long been thoroughly persuaded of the weight and import to mankind of any word he said, that his words really had come to sound as if there were something in them. But now he can only whisper; and what he whispers sounds like what it is - mere jumble and jargon (*BH*, 699/700).

The use of the inarticulate attempt at speech here and its parallel to Anthony Chuzzlewit are obvious, although the social class criticism behind the depiction of Sir Leicester puts a different emphasis on the importance of language. Rather than having abused the power of speech in teaching false values like Chuzzlewit, Sir Leicester has remained silent instead of speaking out to correct social wrongs.

Lord Brain, commenting on the passage above, says "Here is an anticipation of the term 'jargon aphasia'"[16] It is an interesting thought that the person who coined the term may have been familiar with Dickens. The closest I have been able to come to discovering who and when this might have been is Carl Wernicke (1848-1905). He first described the aphasia form bearing his name, of which jargon aphasia is part, in 1874; there is, unfortunately, no evidence whether he was familiar with Dickens.

A little later, Sir Leicester asks for Lady Dedlock and is given her letter, since no one can guess what she wrote. The letter occasions a relapse and, on regaining consciousness an hour later, Sir Leicester wants to write something and can't remember the word. This, too, is typical of certain types of stroke and - as described for Sir Leicester - frustrating and a source of anxiety for patient and caregivers alike:

The slate comes into requisition again; but the word he wants to write, he cannot remember. His anxiety, his eagerness, and affliction at this pass, are pitiable to behold. It seems as if he must go mad, in the necessity he feels for haste, and the inability under which he labours of expressing to do what, or to fetch whom (*BH* 700/01).

Sir Leicester later regains his power of speech, though slowly. He explains his attack to George Rouncewell as

"Something that deadens" - making an endeavour to pass one hand down one side; "and confuses" – touching his lips (*BH*, 729).

This clearly identifies the malady as a stroke, with speech involvement and partial paralysis, though, as usual, Dickens is reticent in giving the malady a name.

We last see Sir Leicester in Lincolnshire, a bent, nearly blind man, but still riding his horse (with George Rouncewell's help) and battling with his neighbour, Boythorn. Though Hillis Miller says that

the stroke which paralyzes Sir Leicester makes him physically what he spiritually has been all along, a frozen and outmoded form of life[17]

one must note that in the one great personal tragedy of Sir Leicester's life, Dickens grants him considerable dignity:

His formal array of words might have at any other time, as it has often had, something ludicrous in it; but at this time it is serious and affecting. His noble earnestness, his fidelity, his gallant shielding of her, his general conquest of his own wrong and his own pride for her sake, are simply honourable, manly, and true (*BH*, 731).

No longer is Sir Leicester the man who utters resounding but meaningless words. He has been transformed in this one short paragraph from an arrogant representative of an "outmoded form of life" to a gentleman in the truest sense of the word. As Peter Gay says:

after his wife flees as her murky past is about to be exposed, this stuffy, reactionary, empty-headed aristocrat shows himself to be a man of authentic decency. He refuses to think ill of the woman who has left him, and keeps hoping – we know that it is in vain – that she will return to him.[18]

The common denominator

It is customary in medicine to speak of "predisposing factors" in the development of a morbid state in the individual patient. Medically, predisposing factors for stroke include smoking, high cholesterol and high blood pressure. The major factor predisposing to stroke for Dickensian characters, however, has revealed itself to be non-medical: his stroke victims are all bad parents or parent figures. The converse does not apply: the majority of the many bad parents/surrogate parents created by Dickens do not suffer stroke – Nell's Grandfather, Paul Dombey, Micawber and a host of others. But the figures discussed here can be seen in three groups: biological parents who neglect or violate their responsibilities (the convict's father, John Willet, Anthony Chuzzlewit, Mrs Skewton, Francis Spenlow,[19] Mrs Steerforth, William Dorrit, Mr Gargery), surrogate parents (Miss Barbary, Mrs Clennam); or parent figures within a paternalistic society (Sir Leicester Dedlock, Josiah Bounderby), who should – and in Dickens's view *must* – bear responsibility for their employees and generally for those less fortunate than themselves. While stroke has been viewed as a punishment, the common denominator has not hitherto been recognised.

Stroke and Dickens himself

The feeling of unconscious prophecy arises in reading both the passage about Francis Spenlow's death and that about Sir Leicester's attack. Dickens's own death is described by Forster as follows:

> he had risen, and his sister-in-law's help alone prevented him from falling where he stood. Her effort was then to get him on the sofa, but after a slight struggle he sank heavily on his left side. "On the ground" were the last words he spoke. . . . All possible medical aid had been summoned. The surgeon of the neighbourhood was there from the first, and a physician from London was in attendance as well as Mr. Beard. But human help was unavailing.[20]

Dickens was not alone at the time of the attack nor did he die quite alone as Francis Spenlow appears to have done. But death was as unexpected for both families. Francis Spenlow reportedly complained of intermittent headache. According to a medical dictionary published in 1829, this could be taken as an early warning sign, along with impaired memory, stammering, dizziness, nightmares, nausea and sensory deceptions.[21] Dickens had had several serious and unequivocal warnings which he chose to ignore despite medical advice. For example, Sir Thomas Watson reported on April 23, 1869 that Dickens had said that "of late [he] sometimes, but rarely, lost or misused a word, that he forgot names or numbers".[22] Here, one may be reminded of Mrs Skewton's missing vocabulary, or her confusing and sometimes mixing the names of her daughter's two husbands, Granger and Dombey, into Grangeby or Domber (*DS*, 602). We must conclude that Dickens knew the danger he was in; his descriptions were too meticulous to let us believe otherwise.[23]

One last curiosity remains to be pointed out in this respect which eerily connects the deaths of Francis Spenlow and Charles Dickens himself. That is the following passage from Chapter 38 *David Copperfield:*

> The shock of such an event happening so suddenly, . . . the appalling vacancy in the room he had occupied so lately, where his chair and table seemed to wait for him, and his handwriting of yesterday was like a ghost - the indefinable impossibility of separating him from the place, and feeling, when the door opened, as if he might come in -. . . (*DC*, 454).

These words conjure up a painting:

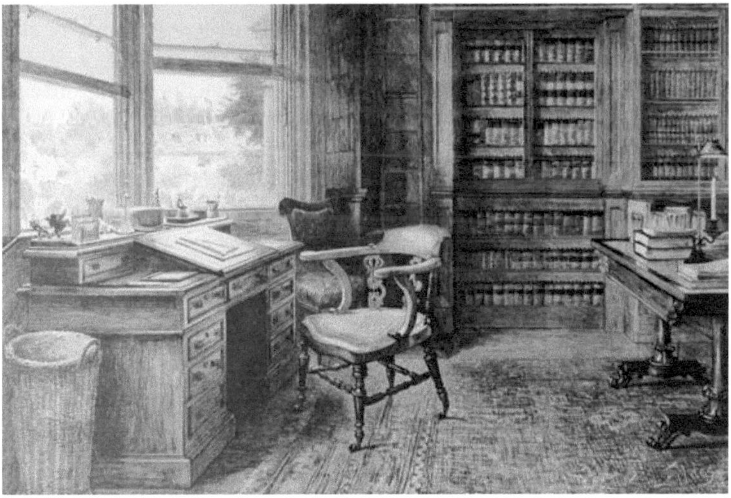

Fig. 6: Fildes, "The Empty Chair." The Dickens Museum.

Conclusion

As we have seen, there are several points to be made concerning the characters in Dickens's work for whom stroke can be postulated. First, one is impressed by the realism of Dickens's descriptions and the way in which he works into his novels various selected aspects of this disorder. Three of the women stroke victims suffer approximately the same debility, with the extent of the insult and the survival time differing slightly. The male victims are more individually characterised, suffering other debilities and surviving for various periods. The fascinating point is that the medical layman Charles Dickens knew of the variations and used them accurately and plausibly, fitting verifiable medical details to the exigencies of his art.

A second point which emerges is that Dickens was aware of the personality changes as well as the physical debility which may be involved in stroke. The truth of his portrait of Mrs Skewton can be attested to by anyone who has cared for stroke victims.

A fascinating point which has apparently not attracted notice to date is the use by Dickens of this disorder as a form of retribution for bad parenting. All of the postulated stroke victims are bad parents/surrogate parents. The poignancy is that this connection can to some extent be applied, unfortunately, to Dickens himself. He was, from all reports, a good father as long as his children were small, but had increasing difficulty relating to them as they grew up.

Stroke was one morbid state which Dickens used in several novels in characters of varying importance. We turn our attention now to another such construct, which, as we will see, again reflects Dickens's knowledge of the disease in its various forms and his genius in using a condition well-known to his reading public to raise awareness of conditions surrounding the disease. This is tuberculosis, a very prevalent disease, affecting up to one-tenth of the nineteenth-century population – which is staging a comeback in new, resistant forms in parts of the world today, often for the same underlying reasons of poverty and deficient sanitation as more than a century ago.

---

[1] *Encyclopaedisches Woerterbuch [EWmW]* 3, 92.

[2] Romans 12:19.

[3] Another such death for literary reasons is seen in Walter Bray, who with his daughter Madeline, was the prototype for William and Amy Dorrit. Bray dies of cardiac arrest rather than stroke.

[4] Forster (1899) I, 166.

[5] Gordon W. Spence in the Introduction to the Penguin Edition of *Barnaby Rudge*, 1973, 14.

[6] Ibid, 19.

[7] Ibid, 25.

[8] Grove (1987), 139.

[9] An earlier pamphlet in response to Sir Andrew Agnew's Sabbath Bill to make a wide variety of activities punishable if carried out on Sunday was published in 1834. Writing under the pseudonym Timothy Sparks, Dickens depicted in "Sunday under Three Heads" Sunday observance "As it is", "As Sabbath Bills would make it" and "As it might be made."

[10] In a July 1857 review of *Little Dorrit* in the *Edinburgh Review*, JF Stephen accused Dickens of using a current news story in the collapse of the house. Dickens's Working Notes, however, make this thread in the story clear from the start.

[11] Engel (1959), 128.

[12] Personal communication, March 4, 1999.

[13] Brain (1955), 126.

[14] This was the original number in Dickens's number plan, but became Chapter 37 in the printed version after Dickens created a new chapter.
[15] Brain (1955), footnote to page 127.
[16] *Ibid*, 128. Interestingly, Brain did not comment on Anthony Chuzzlewit's garbled speech.
[17] Hillis Miller (1958), 220.
[18] Gay (2002), 49.
[19] Spenlow appeared to be a caring father, but it was found that he had left Dora penniless.
[20] Forster (1899), *Life*, II, 511.
[21] *EWmW* 3, 92.
[22] Quoted in Bowen (1956) 147-8.
[23] Prof. I.C. McManus has postulated that Dickens was unaware of the seriousness of his condition. See "Charles Dickens: a neglected diagnosis". *The Lancet* 12, 2001:2158-61. In response, Dr David Bateman of the Royal United Hospital in Bath suggested an alternative neurological diagnosis: premature atherothromboembolic disease and hypertension. *The Lancet* 12, 2002:1253.

CHAPTER 5: Tuberculosis

This chapter deals with the disease Dickens uses most frequently. Three forms of tuberculosis and some of the scenes involving TB victims are discussed. Finally, considerable attention is given to the current status of the medical opinion of certain of these characters to broaden the perspective from which we read these accounts and also to illustrate the interest with which Dickens's works are still read and interpreted by members of the medical profession. It increases our appreciation of Dickens's powers of observation to realize that what, in the past, has been seen as clearly tuberculosis may have been something unknown at the time and only clarified considerably after Dickens's death.

Part of the hypothesis underlying this study is that Dickens's interest in public health would be reflected in his novels. Among the prevalent diseases of the age, the "white plague" or tuberculosis, occupies a special position. Cholera, smallpox, typhoid and typhus caused hundreds of deaths every time they appeared, but they were epidemic. Tuberculosis, by contrast, was omnipresent, killing and crippling thousands every year. It was the single worst disease "cultivated by monster cities..., characterized by fever, night sweats and coughing up blood ... and called 'consumption' because victims were almost literally consumed."[1] The pathogenesis was disputed until the causative organism was identified in 1882 by Robert Koch,[2] but it was recognized that tuberculosis was especially prevalent among the urban poor.

Writing a chapter about tubercular characters in Dickens's works would appear to be a straightforward undertaking. The received medical and lay opinion seems to have been that all of Dickens's crippled and dying children suffered from tuberculosis. Dr A.J. Carter, Consultant Anaesthetist in Stoke-on-Trent who has written articles on Dickens and orthopaedics, reports not having "come across any sick person who did not appear to be suffering from anything other than tuberculosis in one of its many manifestations."[3] The opinion is easily explained, considering the statement in the *British Medical Journal* of January 3, 1857 that "one person in 10 now living will die of [tuberculosis]". There are several forms of the disease which a medical layman might not readily recognize; but they would surely be discussed in medical reviews. This expectation seemed at first to be borne out, but as the adage cited by Fascination Fledgeby in *Our Mutual Friend* [4] has it: things aren't always what they seem. The review of medical journals has revealed that several assumed tuberculosis victims have undergone diagnostic revision, raising some interesting speculations.

Such revisions make apparent the extent to which medical reception has changed over the nearly 100 years since publication of the first article cited in this dissertation. Many common Victorian medical practices have become obsolete, medicine itself has acquired a different form of sophistication, and one might expect that doctors would now deride Dickens's medical descriptions – or perhaps have returned to the earlier habit of simply ignoring them. This is very far from being the case. Rather, differentiated diagnoses of assumedly tubercular figures are still being made. The question is whether the revisions can be substantiated. A search for substantiation not infrequently appears to lead away from the episode in question. It is also in the nature of discourse in medical journals that letters (usually) rebutting the premise appear in subsequent issues. Several such letters are cited to balance the picture. But even when both sides of the present-day medical argument are known, a decision to accept or reject a proposed revision may be made on the basis of the actual text. Where literature and medicine disagree, the reader's own interests and/or way of reading may be expected to tip the scale. Writing as a medical layman, I am aware of my limitations with respect to medical interpretation and diagnosis, but by including the comments and reports of people who are capable of such diagnoses and developing my own interpretation, I may provide a unique perspective.

While most of the deaths found in Dickens's works have been commonly assumed to represent tuberculosis, death will be discussed in this section simply as the natural outcome of the purported disease. Dickens's attitude toward death, his use of death as a literary trope has been thoroughly discussed by Dennis Walder in his book *Dickens and Religion*, particularly Chapter 3.

Forms of the disease

There appear from a lay point of view to be three forms of tuberculosis which Dickens uses. The first is the "fading" form, which claims the most victims. The second most prevalent form in Dickens's works is one that causes crippling, while the third is represented in the novels by one solitary case of painful pulmonary disease.

The "fading" form

This form of tuberculosis was reportedly "by far the most frequent," giving rise to the common lay use of "consumption" as a descriptive term. It was pointed out that in its acute form, death could result within 6-8 weeks, but this was attributed to the probability that the disease only became manifest in a relatively advanced stage.[5] Actually, TB is "a chronic disease, in which the active manifestation may last for years, rather than weeks or months."[6]

There are some interesting observations to be made with respect to this form of tuberculosis in Dickens's works. First, the group ranges from a child of perhaps 8 to a man of indeterminate age. Second, unless we consider Paul Dombey, Junior to be tubercular, all of the figures are to be found in Dickens's "early" works.[7] Third, all of the children are orphans or half-orphans, and all of the people (again except Paul) are poor.

The first figure is found in *Sketches by Boz*, in the last of the "Our Parish" sketches, written in 1835. In "Our Next-Door Neighbours" there is a "young lad of eighteen or nineteen…clothed in deep mourning." He and his mother "were poor – very poor" (46). The boy is described as having "that unearthly light in his plaintive face, which is the beacon of [Nature's] worst disease", and he dies. This "young lad" represents countless victims of the disease and was perhaps based on a real person known to the 23-year-old Dickens. The description is realistic but free from overwhelming pathos; the mother's denial of her son's approaching death and her anguish are simply presented:

> "I was telling William," she said, "that we must manage to take him into the country somewhere, so that he may get quite well." . . . Poor thing! The tears that streamed through her fingers . . . too plainly showed how fruitless was the attempt to deceive herself (*SB*, 46-7).

Dickens has the boy blame life in the city for his demise:

> The boy raised himself by a violent effort, and folded his hands together – "Mother! dear, dear mother, bury me in the open fields – anywhere but in these dreadful streets . . . not in these close crowded streets; they have killed me" (*SB*, 47).

The connection between poverty and disease, especially in cities, had been recognized and was discussed at length during the nineteenth century. Dr William Pulteney Alison, Professor of Medicine in Edinburgh whom Dickens met in 1841 (of whom more is said later in this chapter) was the first to investigate the phenomenon in Scotland. He entered into heated discussions with the theologian Dr Thomas Chalmers concerning the causes of pauperism and the means of combating it. In his reply to Dr Chalmers, Alison quotes W.A. Miles's *Poverty, Mendicity, and Crime*:

> The manufacturing classes in towns, and artisans of most kinds, are much more *subject to disease* than the agricultural population; and there are many employments in themselves unhealthy, and *diseases peculiar to particular trades and callings.*[8]

Dickens, with his experience of the streets of London, had observed the connection and was to comment on it directly and indirectly for the 35 years of his publishing career.

In keeping with the connection of tuberculosis with poverty and privation, the next figure is a Chancery prisoner encountered by Mr Pickwick in the Fleet prison. Pickwick chooses to go to jail rather than pay damages in a trumped-up breach of promise charge brought by Dodson and Fogg for Pickwick's landlady, Mrs Bardell. This gave Dickens chance to use the observations made in his youth when his father, John Dickens, was in jail for debt. It also served as a forum to air the complaint which Dickens raised several times during his career[9] that criminal prisoners were better-treated than honest paupers. We read here, for example, of

> the just and wholesome law which declares that the sturdy felon shall be fed and clothed, and that the penniless debtor shall be left to die of starvation and nakedness (*PP*, 553-4).

Mr Pickwick initially rents a room from the warden, until he learns that, for a price, he can have a room to himself. This he rents from a Chancery prisoner, who "has been consumptive for a long time past."[10] Shortly thereafter, the prisoner dies, having "grown so like death in life, that they knew not when he died" (*PP*, 563).

The third figure in this group is the youngest but one. Oliver Twist's only friend as a small child is an orphan boy named Dick, who was also "farmed" to Mrs Mann. When Oliver runs away from the undertaker, Mr Sowerberry, and heads for London, his path takes him near Mrs Mann's, and Dick is in the garden. Oliver stops to say goodbye, and notes that his friend is very pale. Dick replies:

> I heard the doctor tell them I was dying. … I know the doctor must be right, Oliver, because I dream so much of Heaven, and Angels; and kind faces that I never see when I am awake (*OT*, 43).

Dick dies and Oliver's plans to "take [Dick] away from here, and have him clothed and taught, and send him to some quiet country place where he may grow strong and well" (*OT*, 348) are disappointed.

Oliver's plans for Dick indicate that Dickens was aware of current medical opinion. Dr A.J. Carter sees this knowledge as dating from Dickens's

> first summer holiday at Broadstairs since only 4 miles along the coast, at Margate, an establishment had existed since 1791 to provide London's sick – and especially their children – with the benefits of fresh air.[11]

This institution is the Royal Sea Bathing Hospital, said to be the oldest orthopaedic hospital in the world.

The most famous of Dickens's "fading" tuberculosis victims is Smike, Nicholas Nickleby's cousin. Dr Carter is of the opinion that "Smike's death is absolutely typical of the way these crippled children gradually faded away and died in their teens."[12] The description of the hectic fever attendant on Smike's illness was considered so accurate at the time it was written that it was quoted in full in both Miller's *Principles of Surgery*[13] and Aitken's *The Science and Practice of Medicine.*[14] The description bears some resemblance to that of the Chancery prisoner mentioned above. Also reminiscent of the Chancery prisoner's death: "… a disease in which death and life are so strangely blended, that death takes the glow and hue of life, and life the gaunt and grisly form of death" (*NN*, 637).

Dickens's descriptions of these two figures are, like their fates, similar, but this does not imply that the descriptions are simply part of a stock repertoire of phrases dealing with tuberculosis. It would appear rather that Dickens used parallelism as an identification guide for his readers, since this sort of parallelism in descriptions may be observed in episodes as well as in various characters in different novels. There are similarities, for example, in the descriptions of Mr Gashford (*BR*) and Uriah Heep (*DC*), and in Madeline Bray's self-sacrificing acceptance of marriage to Arthur Gride (*NN*) and Esther Summerson's acceptance of John Jarndyce's proposal (*BH*) (though Madeline's motivation in supporting her father more closely resembles Amy Dorrit's subordination of her own needs).

Susan Sontag uses Smike as an example of the "almost symptomless, unfrightened, beatific deaths from tuberculosis"[15] abounding in nineteenth-century literature. One later statement by Sontag fits Smike also exceptionally well, though Sontag doesn't explicitly make the connection:

> According to the mythology of tuberculosis, there is generally some passionate feeling which provokes, which expresses itself in, a bout of TB. But the passions must be thwarted, the hopes blighted.[16]

The terminal stage of Smike's illness comes after he falls in love with Kate Nickleby and sees her in love with Frank Cheeryble.

The description of Smike's death concurs with recent reports of near-death incidents. Dickens writes:

> [Smike] fell into a light slumber, and waking, smiled as before; then spoke of beautiful gardens, which he said stretched out before him, and were filled with the figures of men, women and many children, all with light upon their faces; then, whispered that it was Eden - and so died (*NN*, 703).

Dr Bruce Greyson of the Department of Psychiatric Medicine, University of Virginia, writes in *The Lancet* of his studies of people reporting such incidents. The article, entitled "Dissociation in people who have near-death experiences: out of their bodies or out of their minds?"[17] classifies such experiences as nonpathological coping mechanisms in the face of stress. This is unlikely in Smike's case. His death was peaceful and accepted as inevitable. The greatest emotional stress he endured toward the end of his life was his unrequited love for Kate, which – compared to what he had endured physically and emotionally at the hands of the brutal schoolmaster, Squeers - was relatively innocuous; but the "vision" was similar not only to what Dick had told Oliver, but also to those reported by Dr Greyson's subjects:

> These experiences . . . include a sensation of being out of the body ... and transcendental elements, such as . . . what is interpreted as an unearthly realm.[18]

Despite early medical appreciation of Dickens's description of tubercular hectic fever, Ann Roulet rates Smike's death as "a real tearjerker. No stock item of a sentimental passing is omitted. . . . It is indeed excessive." [19] While Smike's death is admittedly emotional, "excessive" appears to be a twentieth-century overreaction. The scene fits the general melodrama of the book. *Nicholas Nickleby* is undoubtedly the most theatrical of all of Dickens's novels, (not only because of the Crummleses). Hardly a melodramatic trope is missing: endangered virtue, last-minute rescue, humour, grief, love, hate, villains and heroes are all there. Smike's death is part of this design. Since Dickens's day, death has become largely depersonalised. Dying people are frequently shunted off to hospitals, out of sight of those whom the death might affect emotionally. Surrounded by nurses trained to accept death professionally and "not get involved," a large percentage of people die basically alone. The situation was different in 1839. Not only were people born at home, they also died at home. And young people of Smike's age were frequently victims of tuberculosis, allowing Dickens's contemporary readers to weep over a fictitious death in conscious or unconscious association with experienced death. It would be wrong to disparage the scene because it makes us uncomfortable, which Roulet appears to do. What was a common experience, as well as what was accepted in both medicine and literature when the novel was written, should not be overlooked.

The youngest figure in this group of "fading" deaths appears in *The Old Curiosity Shop*. "He was a very young boy; quite a little child. . . . his eyes were very bright; but their light was of Heaven, not earth" (*OCS*, 200). This could be taken as a foreshadowing of Nell's own death,[20] especially since she tries to hide her grief at the little child's death from her grandfather.

> In the midst of her grief and tears, she was yet careful to conceal their real cause from the old man, for the dead boy had been a grandchild, and left but one aged relative to mourn his premature decay (*OCS*, 201).

After this episode, Nell and her grandfather continue their wanderings, later meeting the same schoolmaster and taking up residence in a cottage next to his.

Nell becomes pale and weakens. "Sometimes . . . the child, exhausted, though with little fatigue, would pass whole evenings on a couch beside the fire" (*OCS*, 425). At one point, a little boy tells her: "They say . . . that you will be an angel, before the birds sing again" (*OCS*, 427). And, in one of the scenes best-known in Dickens's day, her death is reported (the reader is, conspicuously, not present).

Late in the nineteenth century, Oscar Wilde reportedly said that "one must have a heart of stone to read the death of Little Nell without laughing."[21] Quite likely most readers now would agree with Wilde. It must be remembered, however, that nearly half the deaths recorded in London about the time the novel was written were of children less than 10 years of age.[22] Laurence Lerner points out that "the contempt with which twentieth century criticism has dismissed [child deaths] as sentimentalized contrasts vividly with the enthusiasm and tears of contemporaries."[23] Dickens was consciously writing for a public familiar with early deaths and followed a set purpose with the description.[24]

Critics have claimed that in writing of Nell's death, Dickens was obsessed with and reliving the death of his sister-in-law, Mary Hogarth, who died unexpectedly at the age of 17 in 1837 of what is thought to perhaps have been rheumatic heart disease.[25] While it has been argued that Nell was based on Mary Hogarth, the deaths obviously differed. Mary had been entirely well, as far as anyone knew, suddenly collapsed and died on the following day. Nell's impending death was obvious to laymen around her. It would appear logical to ascribe Nell's death to tuberculosis, which was so common at the time the novel was written. But Dr John Cosnett sees the reported joint pains as a sign of rheumatic fever, in which "cardiac complications . . . were among the more common causes of death . . . in the days before penicillin."[26]

In a chronological examination of figures long-considered to have be victims of tuberculosis, we would now turn to the illness and death of little Paul Dombey, who is thought to have been modelled on Dickens's weak, apparently consumptive nephew, Harry Burnett. In my view, however, the "diagnosis" is questionable, so the discussion is put aside for the moment.

The "crippling" form

The second form of tuberculosis used by Dickens is what, for the sake of simplicity, will be termed here "crippling," although this is obviously a layman's oversimplification.

The first "crippled" character is simply incidental to the story. In *Nicholas Nickleby*, Tim Linkinwater's neighbor across the courtyard is a "little hump-backed boy" who must "drag himself about on a pair of tiny crutches" (*NN*,

514). The scene contains a covert hint at Dickens's own childhood: the boy grows flowers in old blacking bottles.

The first major crippled character is the most famous of all: Tiny Tim in *A Christmas Carol.* The Spirit of Christmas Present predicts Tim's death within the coming year and turns Scrooge's Malthusian statement back on him: "If he be like to die, he had better do it, and decrease the surplus population" (*Carol*, 97).

A Christmas Carol illustrates Dickens's understanding of the connection between poverty and disease. "[W]ith *A Christmas Carol*, [Dickens] finally succeeded in awakening the nation's conscience to a problem it had previously been content to ignore."[28] And the effect was lasting: charities were founded for the benefit of crippled children, including one by William Treloar. As a young man, Treloar had heard Dickens read the *Carol* and many years later, as Lord Mayor of London, began a "Lord Mayor's Little Cripple Fund", which opened a home for crippled children in Hampshire in 1908. Now called The Lord Mayor Treloar's Hospital and College, it remains one of Britain's major orthopaedic centres, specialising under the Treloar Trust since 1953 in treatment and education of the disabled. Among the early visitors to the Home was Queen Alexandra, who founded the Alexandra League of Children in 1909 to "encourage the able-bodied to identify with their less fortunate brothers and sisters"[29]- certainly a Dickensian sentiment!

Another major crippled character is found in Dickens's last completed novel, *Our Mutual Friend.* The riverman, Gaffer Hexam, drowns and his daughter, Lizzie, takes lodgings. Her brother, Charley, and the school-master, Bradley Headstone, go to visit Lizzie and find the "person of the house" at home:

> The parlour door within a small entry stood open, and disclosed a child – a dwarf – a girl – a something – sitting on a little low old-fashioned arm-chair …
>
> 'I can't get up,' said the child, 'because my back's bad, and my legs are queer. But I'm the person of the house' (*OMF*, 271).

The child is further described as having a "queer little figure", and a "queer but not ugly little face, with … bright grey eyes" (*OMF*, 272).

That Fanny Cleaver – or Jenny Wren, as she calls herself – has probably been crippled all her life is reflected in her complaint about children:

> Ever so often calling names in through a person's keyhole, and imitating a person's back and legs (*OMF*, 274).

Dickens makes it clear that the children's taunts, coupled with Jenny's lack of a childhood of her own, account for the aggression which she often expresses. As the daughter of a drunken parent in one of Dickens's worst instances of inverted parent-child relationships, Jenny must cope with her own disability and with responsibilities far beyond her years. Until Lizzie Hexam moves into the house, Jenny apparently has no friend or confidante, and it is Lizzie's womanly presence that lets Jenny mature emotionally. Her nature, outwardly vengeful and malicious, is in fact capable of the best (in Dickens's opinion) womanly traits. Apparently a natural nurse,[30] she helps tend Eugene Wrayburn after the brutal attack by Headstone, and it appears implied that Jenny will eventually marry the young man known only as "Sloppy".

The "gasping" form

The one case of death from painful pulmonary disease is Jo, the crossing sweeper in *Bleak House.* He infects Charley and Esther with smallpox and – taken away by Inspector Bucket to a "horsepittle" – disappears from the narrative. When he reappears, he is seen by Jenny, the brickmaker's wife, and Allan Woodcourt. Jo is obviously ill and says that he is dying. His breath, he says "'draws as heavy as a cart.' He might add, 'and rattles like it'" (*BH*, 584). The metaphor of the cart is maintained through to Jo's death.

> For the cart so hard to draw, is near its journey's end, and drags over stony ground. All round the clock it labours up the broken steps, shattered and worn. Not many times can the sun rise, and behold it still upon its weary road (*BH*, 594).

Bleak House was the first novel written since Dickens's sister, Fanny's, death. It would appear that Dickens was using the observations he made at the time. He had written to Kate at the end of August 1848 that "[n]o words can express the terrible aspect of suffering and suffocation – the appalling noise in [Fanny's] throat – and the agonizing look around."[31] That he equated this "appalling noise" with the sound of a heavy cart being dragged over stony ground seems plausible and might explain why this form of the disease occurs in this particular novel.

Most books attribute Fanny's death to tuberculosis, but there is one dissenting diagnosis on record. Dr Norman Jacoby writes in "Charles Dickens' Asthma" that he finds no convincing evidence that the diagnosis of tuberculosis in Fanny is correct, and goes on to point out that

> by good fortune, after Fanny's death, Dickens' fear that tuberculosis would continue to ravage the family proved unfounded, and makes it highly improbable that in her case it was a true bill. It can hardly be overstressed that asthma in its own right can be a fatal disease.[32]

This does not, however, alter my opinion that Dickens was using his own observations, even if the disease was not what he thought.

That would complete the review of conspicuous characters commonly assumed to have suffered tuberculosis in the works of Dickens. But medicine has not stood still and three of the most famous of Dickens's afflicted children have been "rediagnosed". They were not questioned in the order of their creation; the first was Paul Dombey in 1984; the second Tiny Tim in 1992; and the last Jenny Wren in 1996 and again in 1999.

In 1984, Howard Markel writing in "Charles Dickens and the Art of Medicine" cites, as one example of disease in Dickens's works, "an excellent description of acute lymphocytic leukaemia in young Paul Dombey of *Dombey and Son.*" [33] This quite contradicts the usual view, reflected for example in a statement by Dr Paul G. Jones of the Royal Children's Hospital in Melbourne. In a lecture delivered in Adelaide in 1971, Dr Jones stated:

> Paul was ... pale, wan and weakly at 5 years of age, but Paul improved sufficiently to go to Dr Blimber's School . . . until he wasted and died. These details, too [like those of Tiny Tim] are somewhat meagre but a remission of nearly 2 years, if such it was, would rule out leukaemia ...[34]

Markel undoubtedly knew of this problem, but he presents considerable support for his hypothesis. In Markel's opinion, the diagnosis seems likely from the description: the child was pale, anorexic, increasingly weak, highly susceptible to infections, and he suffered pain in his bones.

Markel's hypothesis undoubtedly has some grave drawbacks from a medical point of view. But what of a literary point of view? Here it would seem reasonable to give Markel's opinion serious consideration. To begin with, Dickens was using a totally new approach in writing about Paul Dombey. This early appearance of what has become stream of consciousness writing is not a first-person narrative. The child is neonate at the beginning of the book and dies in the fifth number of twenty, so using Paul as a first-person narrator would have been difficult. But the reader does see much of what Paul is experiencing through his eyes. It is he who reports the fatigue and aching bones:

> Florence is older than I am, but I'm not as strong and well as Florence. . . . I am so tired sometimes . . . and my bones ache so . . . that I don't know what to do (*DS*, 100).

The onset of the terminal phase of Paul's illness is described as experienced:

> But there seemed to be something the matter with the floor, for he couldn't stand upon it steadily; and with the walls, too, for they were inclined to turn round and round, . . . Paul observed with astonishment that the door was in quite a different place from that in which he had expected to find it and almost thought, at first, that Mr Toots was going to walk straight up the chimney (*DS*, 201).

There is nothing here on which to base a diagnosis. The description could be tuberculosis, leukaemia – or any one of a number of even minor things associated with weakness and dizziness. Laurence Lerner postulates, for example, that Paul might have had asthma.[35] But, writes Lerner, "who can doubt that Paul died of consumption . . ."[36] Doubt is, however, possible. It might be asked whether Dickens, using a new approach, was also using a new disease?

Formerly, the answer would have been that there was no need to use anything new. The purpose of the novel was to "do with Pride what its predecessor [*MC*] had done with Selfishness." [37] Tuberculosis was the scourge of childhood. Seeing his son die of a disease that indiscriminately killed thousands would be severely humiliating for Paul Dombey, Senior, denying him any possible comfort afforded by the thought that it took something new and unknown to kill his son, a thought which his pride could perhaps have fastened on as setting a Dombey apart, even in death.

Diagnostic speculations

The phrase "new and unknown" raises an historical question: was leukaemia known when *Dombey* was written? A search for the answer to that question led to some interesting facts – and to some speculation. To start: leukaemia was first described in 1845. *Dombey* was begun in late June 1846, publication started in October 1846, with Paul's death in the fifth number, published in January 1847. So leukaemia *was*, in fact, known; at least the first articles had been published.

The name generally associated with the discovery of leukaemia is the "father of pathological anatomy" Rudolf Virchow (1821-1902),[38] at the time working at the Charité Hospital in Berlin. What frequently escapes attention is the article published in Edinburgh by John Hughes Bennett (1812-1875) about 5 months *before* Virchow's article appeared.[39] The first banquet in Dickens's honour was held in Edinburgh in 1841. Might Dickens have met Hughes Bennett then? K.J. Fielding, in his collection of Dickens's *Speeches*, makes no mention of Hughes Bennett in connection with the banquet, nor however of the "Dr Alison" whom Dickens himself mentioned to Forster, as "a very popular friend of the poor."[40] Dickens also told Forster of an invitation: "Monday, dine at Dr Alison's, four miles off." But there is no closer identification of Dr Alison.

Further investigation into Hughes Bennett and leukaemia provided more support for the speculation that Dickens and Hughes Bennett may have been acquainted – and incidentally identified Dr Alison. Dr Gordon Piller published an article entitled "John Hughes Bennett, His Life and the Identification of Leukaemia." A picture of professors at Edinburgh in about 1850 shows, among others James Miller (surgery), James Young Simpson (midwifery) [41] as well as John Hughes Bennett (institutes of medicine) and William Pulteney Alison (medicine). Alison's interest in the connection between disease and poverty mentioned above obviously motivated his inviting Dickens to dinner. By 1841, Dickens's reputation as a champion of the poor was already fairly well-established. The first collected *Sketches* had been published in 1836 with individual sketches published in 1835; *The Pickwick Papers* (1836-37), with the scenes of destitute debtors in the Fleet; *Oliver Twist* (1837-39) with its biting criticism of the New Poor Law; *Nicholas Nickleby* (1838-39) exposing Yorkshire schools and the plight of milliners were known; and *The Old Curiosity Shop*, depicting poverty among mill workers, had been completed only the January previous to the banquet. We need certainly look no further. But can we assume that Hughes Bennett was also invited to dinner that evening? This might appear justified.

Piller rounds his article off with some biographical information about Hughes Bennett, and here we find some clues. Hughes Bennett's father, John Bennett, was a distinguished musician and comedy actor, who married Julia Hughes. Julia's father was Richard Hughes, who owned not only the Theatre Royal in Exeter, but also Sadler's Wells Theatre in London. The plausible link in the association of London – theatre – Dickens is conspicuous. Moreover, Hughes Bennett's uncle was the clown, Joseph Grimaldi. Dickens had been taken as a child to see Grimaldi perform[42] and in 1837 had been asked by Richard Bentley to edit Grimaldi's memoirs. The book was published in February 1838.[43] If we assume that Alison knew this, mightn't we assume also that he would invite his young colleague to meet the author?

Piller writes that Hughes Bennett had completed his studies in Edinburgh, gone for two years post-graduate training to Paris, followed by ten months in Germany, including six months at the Charité. "By summer of 1841, Bennett was back in Edinburgh."[44] The banquet was held on June 25, a Friday. Since Dickens and Kate arrived on June 23 and left Edinburgh on July 4 for a tour of the Highlands,[45] dinner "Monday evening" must have been on June 28. Is that summer? Dr Piller, in a reply to a specific inquiry, expressed doubts that "Bennett met Dickens in 1841 because at that time, he was re-establishing himself in Edinburgh in academic medicine and might have arrived later than did Dickens."[46] The hypothesis is not necessarily rejected. Bennett was not "establishing" himself as a stranger. He had been an outstanding student during the four years he spent reading medicine. His dissertation on "Physiology and Pathology of the Brain" had been deemed worthy of a gold medal (but he had already been awarded one for the best clinical report of surgical cases, and the rules disallowed more than one to any one student).[47] Alison had been teaching in Edinburgh since 1818, taking the Chair in Pathology and Physiology in 1820; Bennett began reading medicine in Edinburgh in 1833. The two were most certainly acquainted. Unfortunately, the dinner invitation remains speculation, since apparently no records have survived. There is also little correspondence known between Alison and Dickens, with none before 1846, and none between Bennett and Dickens.

Dr Piller also rejects the possibility of leukaemia as a diagnosis for Paul, but widens the discussion by postulating coeliac disease. If correct, it would be one of several instances of Dickens's anticipating medical science. Piller writes:

> The symptoms that Dickens describes, albeit briefly, could point to a diagnosis of coeliac disease, a condition not recognized until 1952 which if untreated would result in death within 5 years of birth. My discussions with medical colleagues confirm this view and we are told by Dickens that Paul died at about the age of 5. [48]

This theory self-destructs in the last sentence. Paul was six when he left Mrs Pipchin's. Mr Dombey decides to have him attend Dr Blimber's boarding school, and notes that the child is "getting on" and is all of "six years old" (*DS*, 147). Since Paul "goes home for the holidays" at the end of the school year, never to return, he must have been about seven then and died somewhere near the age of eight.

The factors contributing to Piller's opinion are confirmed in *Harrison's Principles of Internal Medicine*. Patients with coeliac disease, or non-tropical sprue, may complain of bone pain. Treatment for this disease is now known to be a gluten-free diet, whereby if the patient does not respond to diet, "he or she may have developed intestinal lymphoma."[49] This could mean that the discussion has come a full circle: Paul was not created as a tuberculosis victim. But some form of cancer may have been depicted, if not leukaemia as such.

A second article in the supplementary volume on John Hughes Bennett adds a few more curiosities to the discussion. In his article "Suppuration of the Blood: The Biology of Leukaemia, Past, Present and Future." D.J. Weatherall writes:

> During the first 100 years after its discovery, many infection agents were suggested as candidates for the cause of leukaemia, notably *tuberculosis* and malaria [my emphasis].
>
> The bone marrow in leukaemia has many features of pernicious anaemia.[50]

This, again, takes us back to Piller via *Harrison's*: "a [sprue] patient may be admitted for investigation of iron deficiency anaemia ..."

Criticism of the leukaemia "diagnosis"

As predicted above, this has led away not only from the episode, but also from Markel's original article and the criticism it received. Dr A.L. Freedman replied in a letter to the editor concerning several points in connection with leukaemia. Freedman was unconvinced by Markel's arguments first because of the length of time the child was ill, which he calculates as about twenty months. Second, Freedman opinion's is that "an artist with a palette like Dickens' would not have failed to mention the purpura, epistaxis and lymphadenopathy that are expected in patients dying of acute lymphatic leukaemia." He then cites several possibilities – not only bovine tuberculosis, but also severe anaemia. He concludes that "The prime diagnosis, however, is that Paul died a literary death, wasting and pining sweetly away for the benefit of author and reader." [51]
This latter diagnosis is the only one guaranteed correct. But having plausibly overcome the objection that leukaemia wasn't known, counterarguments can be raised. Taking Freedman's objections in order, it can be argued as follows:

The child was sick too long. This is known *now*, but was it when the novel was written? The original description of the disease was based on autopsy cases: Virchow's a fifty-year-old woman, Bennett's a twenty-eight-year-old man. But what details were known prior to autopsy? These cases would at any rate appear to be different than acute leukaemia in a six-year-old child.

A literary reason for the course of the disease must be taken into account, especially remembering Freedman's "prime diagnosis". In a letter to Forster, Dickens wrote: "I hope you will like Mrs Pipchin's establishment. It is from the life, and I was there –"[52] Edgar Johnson says: "Mrs Pipchin was in fact a fusion of the old woman who kept a dame-school at Chatham and Mrs Roylance of the Bayham Street days."[53] Forster tells us that Dickens "was a very little and a very sickly boy."[54] How much of the stream-of-consciousness approach Dickens used for Paul Dombey may be drawn from subconscious – or even conscious – recollection would perhaps be an interesting speculation. Suffice it here, however, to note the possibility, especially in conjunction with the memory of Mrs Roylance.

Freedman's objection that *Dickens would not have failed to mention the purpura, epistaxis and lymphadenopathy that are expected in patients dying of acute lymphatic leukaemia* raises another medical-historical question: had these signs already been identified in relation to the underlying disease? Even so, it cannot be concluded that Dickens "failed to mention" them. All that can be definitively said is that he *didn't* mention them. This, however, must be viewed in light of what was considered "proper" at the time the novel was written. Dickens could not have included physical details in his description.

Another counterargument here is the narrative perspective. While a six-year-old boy might talk about nosebleeds (epistaxis), it is not likely that he would have much to say about swollen glands (lymphadenopathy/Hodgkin's disease) or bleeding under the skin (purpura). Such physical details would also not be probable for Paul as he is depicted. A "quaint, old-fashioned child," who listens to what the waves are saying and thinks about dying "on a moonlight night, when the sky was quite clear and the wind blowing" (*DS*, 180) would not be likely to occupy his thoughts with the purely – and unpleasantly – physical.

That Paul is sent to Brighton has been taken as "proof" that he was tubercular, in light of the importance of Brighton as a spa prior to the 1840s. It is well, however, to remember that *Dombey* is 1840s Dickens and not 1870s Eliot. That is, Dickens's doctors were men of the healing *art* and not men of science, like Eliot's Dr Lydgate. It is questionable whether Dr Peps and Mr Pilkins possessed a microscope – prerequisite to diagnosing leukaemia. Assuming they did not, the most likely diagnosis, given Paul's symptoms and the medical environment in which the novel was written, would be bovine tuberculosis. The doctors would then have sent the child to Brighton, with the resultant lack of therapeutic success.

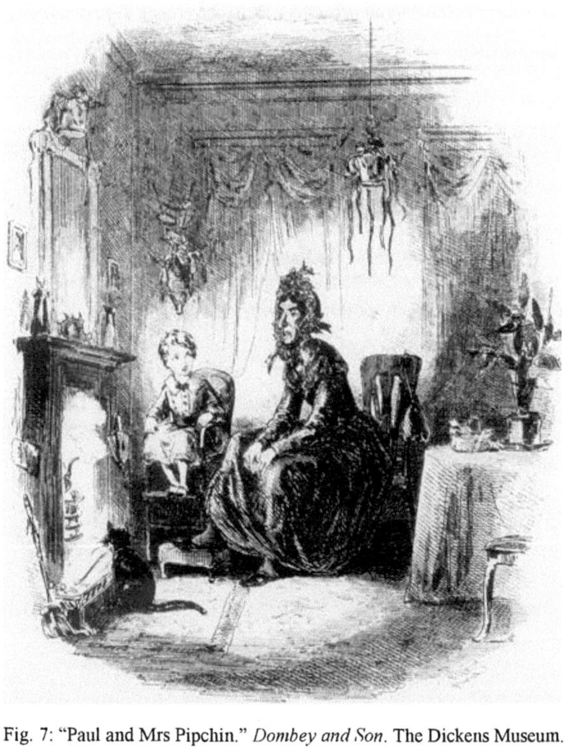

Fig. 7: "Paul and Mrs Pipchin." *Dombey and Son*. The Dickens Museum.

Taking these facts and speculations together, Markel's opinion would seem to gain in plausibility. Perhaps Paul Dombey really is the first literary victim of leukaemia

Alternative diagnoses

There is at least one other possibility, which might be medically more acceptable in its entirety today. It can be postulated that Paul's complaint was rheumatic heart disease. This would account for the fainting and weakness due to lack of oxygen to the tissues, the damaged valves would produce clots which, breaking off, would cause ministrokes. Remembering that the main contrast in this novel of contrasts is that between the deaths of Paul and Mrs Skewton,[57] it is interesting to consider that Dickens may have let the characters die of similar causes. The main objection to rheumatic heart disease is that it does not affect very young children, but rather adolescents and young adults like Mary Hogarth. A congenital heart defect would thus be more likely and would produce the outcome described.

Assuming Paul's death to be due to some form of heart disease would also tie in with the clock theme used at Paul's birth and again at his death. The association of doctors and watches can be viewed in several ways. On the one hand, there is the association between time as life at Paul's birth and its contrast time as death in the same scene in connection with Mrs Dombey and later with Paul himself. On the other hand, watches have a rhythmic function, ticking steadily to mark the passage of time, thus being a metaphor for the heart. At the time Dickens was writing, heart rate, expressed in "beats per minute," was one of the few measures of cardiac function available to the doctor. The image of the doctor feeling his patient's pulse is ingrained in the lay conscience, as Captain Cuttle demonstrates when Florence runs from her father to the Wooden Midshipman and faints. She begins to regain consciousness and

> At this stage of her recovery, Captain Cuttle, with an imperfect association of a Watch with a Physician's treatment of a patient, took his own down from the mantel-shelf, and holding it out on his hook, and taking Florence's hand in his, looked steadily from one to the other, as expecting the dial to do something (*DS*, 707).

The association between the heart and a timepiece is also conspicuous at Dr Blimber's, where the grandfather clock on the stairs keeps saying "how-is-my-lit-tle-friend". It is not impossible that Dickens was subtly pointing to a cardiac disease in thus connecting Paul with the grandfather clock.

As interesting as the speculation around leukaemia is, and though the by-ways into which the speculation have led have brought to light details which could support the "diagnosis," it would appear more likely that Dickens had some sort of congenital heart disease in mind when he created Paul Dombey. Certainly a morbid state somehow related to the stroke described for Mrs Skewton would fit better into the pattern of contrasts around which the novel is constructed.

Revision among the "crippled" victims

The next assumed tuberculosis victim with revised diagnosis is Tiny Tim in *A Christmas Carol.* Tim's illness has received more attention from the medical world than that of any other single character. Not only have there been more articles, but the response to the articles has also been greater. Markel's article cited above brought one published letter discussing only one of the diseases mentioned. Articles on Tim have brought numerous published responses and reportedly a veritable flood of mail to the authors.

As discussed above, A.J. Carter includes Tim in his discussion of Dickens's crippled children, who were all – in Carter's opinion – victims of tuberculosis. The diagnosis for Tim reached by Paul G. Jones was also that the most likely disease was tuberculosis of the hip, or "coxalgia."[58] This "carried with it a sentence of gross deformity and frequently death – as foreshadowed by the Ghost of Christmas Present." Jones surmises, however, that Tim's recovery would suggest Perthes' disease, which would be another Dickensian diagnosis in anticipation of medical science, since "that particular diagnosis was still 77 years away in the future (Calvé, 1910)." [59]

Donald W. Lewis of the Department of Pediatric Neurology in Virginia used the case of Tiny Tim as a teaching tool. While Lewis admits that the case as presented is vague, the "patient" was well known to the class participants and the task of "diagnosis" was enthusiastically undertaken. Unlike many of the doctors publishing retrospective diagnoses for Dickens's characters, Lewis begins by asking:

> What disease processes might have been recognized or treatable in Dickens' London of 1843? Can the usual problem-solving techniques be used to generate a differential diagnosis in the attempt to settle on a single plausible explanation? [60]

The "diagnostic" points agreed on are as follows:

1. Tim is crippled

   Alas for Tiny Tim, he bore a little crutch, and had his limbs supported by an iron frame (*Carol,* 94).

2. He is of stunted growth

He is "Tiny" Tim; and his younger brother and sister "hustled Tiny Tim, and bore him off to the wash-house, that he might hear the pudding singing in the copper" (*Carol,* 94), so younger siblings could carry him.

3. The disease which cripples Tim will kill him within a year.

If these shadows remain unaltered . . ., none other of my race [The Christmas Spirits] … will find him here (*Carol,* 97).

4. The disease is reversible

Tiny Tim, who did NOT die… (*Carol,* 133).

Before revealing the conclusion reached, Lewis rules out some common possibilities. Discussion included congenital syphilis (ruled out since Tim is not mentally retarded) and even child abuse (also ruled out, since the Cratchits are one of the extremely few functional families in Dickens's works). Scurvy, described by the Scottish naval surgeon, James Lind (1716-1794) in 1753, is considered unlikely, since the family consume potatoes and lemons. Rickets, prevalent enough to be called "the English disease," had been found by investigators by mid-century to be reversible by means of cod-liver oil, and is also considered unlikely, since Tim was apparently the only family member afflicted.

Reviewing mid-nineteenth century paediatric texts, Lewis notes that "[a]ir, exercise, and proper nourishment are, in these cases, our chief remedial agents." [61] Tim's crippling skeletal disorder would, says Lewis, have "directed clinicians toward the treatment of tuberculosis." Another mid-century text[62] points out that both rickets and tuberculosis were to be treated with the same methods. Both texts postulated the presence of excessive acid in scrofula patients and prescribed a 'prudent' dose of alkaline carbonates, such as bicarbonate of soda, to combat the hyperacidity. This leads Dr Lewis to the assumption of the following regimen for Tim: "Fresh air and sunshine, a balanced diet, . . . cod-liver oil, and mineral waters or tonics emphasizing alkaline solutions with bitters." From this, he concludes that the tonics and solutions are the key to the diagnosis and reversibility of Tim's disease, since "alkaline solutions . . . and Vitamin D remain today the treatment for renal tubular acidosis (RTA)." [63] Lewis points out that the disease was not recognized until the early twentieth century by Albright Lightwood, and that the clinicians in the 1840s would not have known what they were actually treating, but as "keen empiricists, they would have recognized the beneficial effects of the aforementioned regimen."[64]

Responses to Lewis's article appeared in the *American Journal of Diseases of Children* in August 1993. Dr Russell Chesney, Department of Pediatrics, University of Tennessee[65] raises several points against the diagnosis, among them that the disease postulated by Lewis is often – though not exclusively -

hereditary, and there is no evidence that Bob or Mrs Cratchit was affected. Also, Dr Chesney doubts a lethal outcome for RTA. He sees a greater statistical probability in either polio or tuberculosis.

Dr Douglas Peterson [66] postulates other reasons why Tim might have died in the coming year – all of them directly due to poverty and environmental factors. As Winnifred J. Pederson points out in connection with Jo of *Bleak House*, Dickens is aware "that the environment has an inescapable effect on the development of people."[67] This may, indeed, have been the explanation of Tim's anticipated demise.

Interesting as Dr Lewis's article is, there are reasons to doubt his conclusions. Several of the "diagnostic data" appear to have been misread. First, Dr Lewis apparently overemphasises the alliterative "Tiny Tim." It must be remembered that several of Dickens's figures both before and after the *Carol* were called "little," of whom Little Dorrit was the only one so slight that she was taken for a child although she was 20. "Little" is a term of endearment and one which evokes sympathy and pity. "Tiny" has even greater power to evoke these emotions, which Dickens consciously applied.

Lewis postulates that Tim suffered from intermittent weakness, but this he concludes only from Tim's being carried home from church. Lewis has apparently overlooked Bob's preparations for leaving Scrooge's counting house on Christmas Eve:

> The office was closed in a twinkling, and the clerk, with the long ends of his white comforter dangling below his waist (for he boasted no great-coat), went down a slide on Cornhill, at the end of a lane of boys, twenty times, in honour of its being Christmas-eve (*Carol*, 53).

Bob was supporting his family of eight on 15 "bob" a week. He had no coat, and probably his children were also inadequately dressed against the cold. There was snow on the ground, making progress slower than usual for a crippled boy. It would be logical for a parent to carry the child under such circumstances, if only to get him inside as quickly as possible.

Later in the text, the phrase "bore him off" need not be read to mean that Tim's brother and sister literally *carried* him to hear the pudding singing in the copper. One can be "borne off" by the power of persuasion – and Tim probably needed little persuasion to increase his anticipation of the once-yearly treat.

Dr Lewis makes other statements which do not appear to be supported by the *Carol* itself. For instance, there is no original illustration depicting Tim, so Lewis is relying on film-makers or musical directors for the "fact" that the

disease was reversible. Dickens did not say this. "Tiny Tim did NOT die" does not necessarily mean that the child became perfectly healthy. There is a linguistic difference between "stop" and "reverse" which applies medically as well.
There was also an article published in *The Dickensian* on the subject in 1993: "Tiny Tim: The Child with a Crippling Fatal Illness." Dr Charles W. Callahan of the US Army Medical Center in Honolulu ponders which of several diseases may have been responsible and concludes that

> There is one type of chronic but deadly infection which was so prevalent in Dickens's era that it would easily have provided inspiration for his character of Tiny Tim.

Callahan considers Pott's disease, a form of tuberculosis first described by the London surgeon Percival Pott (1713-1788) in 1779; or agrees with the article by Paul Jones cited above, that coxalgia is a plausible explanation. Callahan concludes with a statement which applies not only to Tim, but – unfortunately – to nearly this entire study: "It is, of course, impossible to know exactly what Charles Dickens had in mind."[68]

An article appeared in the *Washington Post* on December 24, 2002 based essentially on the articles by Lewis and Callahan. Roxanne Nelson, a free-lance writer, also interviewed the doctors, who defended their positions: Callahan maintains that

> Fresh air, good nutrition and rest, along with a custom-fitted back brace, could have helped halt the progression of [Tim's] disease or even put him into remission.

Lewis, on the other hand, defends his claim of complete healing, saying:

> You have to buy into the essence of the story. Something happens to Tim physiologically which heals him, and that is a parallel to Scrooge's spiritual rebirth.[69]

Malcolm Andrews, who was also contacted by Ms Nelson, sees the discussion as largely irrelevant, since "Dickens was not concerned about being 'clinically' specific and . . . Tim's suffering is metaphorical."[70] But medical evidence strongly supports the assumption that Dickens *was* concerned about being clinically *correct*. While this does not affect the message of the fable, it may explain why clinicians more than a century and a half later still find it fascinating to examine the evidence. As in daily practice, the doctors put aside the *human* implications of the story and try to make sense of the medical details.

Like the majority of commentators in medical journals – and indeed apparently of all commentators since publication of the *Carol* – I remain of the opinion that

Tiny Tim was most likely created as a victim of tuberculosis. This disease killed and maimed so many hundreds of thousands and was so prevalent at the time Dickens was writing that it would have served his purpose like no other. Anything which cripples or kills a child would rouse sympathy, but for nineteenth-century readers, tuberculosis had an ever-present actuality which should not be underestimated. The overwhelming point is that 160 years after his creation, Tim is still able to move people to the response intended by Dickens: How can we help? What can and must be done to prevent the death of this child and others like him?

Jenny Wren

The final character to undergo diagnostic revision is Fanny Cleaver, or Jenny Wren, the doll's dressmaker, in *Our Mutual Friend,* who has been assigned at least two divergent diagnoses.

Writing in *The Pharos* in 1996, Dr James Gamble discusses the living conditions in mid-Victorian Britain, including the working-class diet and air pollution, which both contributed to the prevalence of rickets. The disease, in which there is characteristic outward curvature of the lower leg bones, had been described in 1645 by Daniel Whistler (1619-1684).[71] A classic clinical description written by Francis Glisson (1597-1677) in 1650 describes rachitic children as being "for the most part of forward wits," in whom "some bones wax crooked... from hence it comes to pass that some Children long afflicted with this Disease become Dwarfs."[72] From Dickens's description of Jenny, Dr Gamble concludes that her deformity is consistent with "patients who had rickets, but not . . . patients with . . . juvenile rheumatoid arthritis, . . . syphilis or fetal alcohol syndrome." Gamble also notes that "at that time about 10 percent of rachitic patients had scoliosis, or curvature of the spine," which would account for Jenny's "bad back." Scoliosis is implied in Jenny's description of herself as being "awfully lopsided".[73]

Contrary to the explicit rejection of foetal alcohol syndrome in Dr Gamble's article, Dr John Cosnett, in a letter to the editor of *Addiction,* points out the numerous characters in Dickens's works who were chronic alcoholics, including Jenny's father and grandfather. Dr Cosnett writes

> This reference to [Jenny's] father and grandfather being addicted to alcohol indicates that Dickens knew of a familial association in this malady, a century before twin and adoption studies have shown a definite hereditary influence.[74]

Dr Cosnett goes on to speculate that Jenny's mother was perhaps also alcoholic, since, unlike Dr. Gamble, he sees in Jenny an example of foetal alcohol syndrome (FAS). This syndrome, in which there are stunted growth and facial peculiarities, could be implied in Dickens's description of Jenny (see above). Her "queer legs" could also be part of the syndrome. Dr Cosnett does allow that Jenny is normally intelligent and that the "remarkable dexterity of her nimble fingers" would not support the diagnosis. However, possibly Jenny's mother was not constantly in the habit of drunkenness, but a "binge drinker," resulting in an incomplete syndrome; or perhaps Dickens used as much of the syndrome which he observed as was consistent with the character he wished to create.

Today's FAS is certainly plausible. But there are other possibilities which would not malign Jenny's mother, since her being married to an alcoholic doesn't necessarily make her one as well. Polio would be possible, for example, in Jenny's case. Or her debility might also result from child abuse by a drunken father – a possibility also cited by Dr Gamble.

The facial characteristics of FAS – very thin, almost invisible upper lip, wide space between nose and mouth and flattened bridge of the nose – are not shown in Marcus Stone's two illustrations of Jenny full-face or in profile. Dickens was less particular by 1865 in his instructions to his illustrators than he had been, certainly, but since he mentioned Jenny's face, it was obviously important to his perception of her, and it surprises somewhat that there is no reflection in the illustrations.

Dr Cosnett admits that Jenny may have had tuberculosis of one or even both hips, causing her mobility problems, but prefers a single diagnosis, where there is one that will fit, to a combination of diagnoses. He also warns about assuming that just because a disease is common, every disease which appears at all similar must be that disease.[75] This is contrary to the opinion expressed by Dr Douglas Peterson in responding to Dr Lewis's article on Tiny Tim: "When you hear hoofbeats, think of horses. Common things are common." And while "things aren't always what they seem, they usually are!"[76] After reviewing the various texts, I find Dr Gamble's diagnosis of rickets the most likely, since it eliminates the need to postulate incomplete syndromes and fits Jenny's own description of herself.

Conclusion

This review of the apparently tubercular characters in Dickens's works reinforces our appreciation of Dickens's powers of observation and description. Dickens uses a prevalent disease in a variety of its manifestations in novels ranging from the fairy-tale/allegory ambience of *The Old Curiosity Shop* to the realism of *Our Mutual Friend.* Consistent with its occurrence at the time, tuberculosis is the disease claiming the greatest number of victims among Dickensian characters – even when those who no longer appear unequivocally tubercular are subtracted from the total.

The "model" for the characters is debatable, with only Jo's disease in *Bleak House* traceable to Dickens's biography. The correlation between Dickens's correspondence at the time of Fanny's death and the description of Jo's death in *Bleak House* has not, however, been noted in any of the articles consulted for this dissertation. The other characters would appear to have been created out of Dickens's imagination based on observations outside his family. The disease was certainly to be observed, by those who did not look away. Dickens, greatly concerned by the relationship between poverty and disease, aimed in his writings to make people see what they otherwise chose to ignore. Tuberculosis attained a certain romantic aura not associated with other diseases, and Dickens was able to capitalise on that aura while protesting against unsanitary conditions, overcrowding, inadequate diet and other detrimental influences of poverty. As pointed out in a recent commentary by Gro Harlem Bruntland, director-general of the World Health Organization, and James D. Wolfensohn, president of the World Bank, tuberculosis is resurgent in much of the world and "the emergence of drug-resistant strains has revived the centuries-old reputation of tuberculosis as the 'Captain of Death'". The disease still "thrives on poverty and social disruption." [77] So, although the possibility of treatment has improved, the underlying factors have not changed since Dickens's day.

We now turn our attention to a disease used in a single novel, but used to a degree otherwise not apparent in Dickens's medical episodes. This is smallpox, which Dickens used in a particularly potent way to connect several of the themes addressed in *Bleak House.*

---

[1] Porter (1997), 401.

[2] *Harrison's*, 700. Robert Koch (1843-1910), German bacteriologist.

[3] Personal communication, January 29, 1999.

[4] *OMF*, Book II, Ch. 5.

[5] *Enzyklopaedisches Wörterbuch der medicinischen Wissenschaften [EWmW]*, 27 (1842), 247.

[6] Hardy, 1993, 212.

[7] The "early works" are those preceding *DS.* Paul's "diagnosis" will be discussed later. Including him would only extend the range to the first of the "middle" novels and thus have no significant impact on this statement.

[8] Alison (1841). Original italics.

[9] See also *David Copperfield,* Chapter 61; and "Fat Convicts", *All the Year Round,* March 25, 1865. Detailed information is found in Collins, *Dickens and Crime* (1982) and Chapter 6, fn 28, 236 below.

[10] This is the only one of Dickens's TB victims in whom the disease is specified, but Dr Cosnett points out that the term was applied to many chronic wasting diseases (Cosnett, 2003), 24.

[11] Carter (1993), 45-48.

[12] Carter, personal communication January 29, 1999. Carter places Smike in the "crippled" group. It appears, however, that Dickens distinguished between "lame" and "crippled" and that Smike's lameness is therefore just as likely due to abuse by Squeers.

[13] Miller, (1850), 46.
[14] Aitkin (1866), 111.
[15] Sontag (1979) 16.
[16] *Ibid*, 22.
[17] *The Lancet*, 355, February 5, 2000, 460-3.
[18] Greyson (2000), 461.
[19] Roulet (1964), 122.
[20] Little Nell's death is discussed in Chapter 1.
[21] Quoted in Malcolm Andrews's Introduction to the Penguin edition of *The Old Curiosity Shop* (1972), 27.
[22] Dudgeon (1987), 139.
[23] Lerner (1997).
[24] See his speech in Edinburgh, June 25, 1841, in: Fielding.(1988), 10.
[25] Mary's younger brother, George, died under similar circumstances a few years later, so there appears to have been an inherited cardiac complaint. No autopsy was done in either case and the cause remains speculation.
[26] Cosnett (2003), 23.
[27] Forster, *Life*, I, 22. *Nicholas Nickleby* was written 1838-1839.
[28] Carter (1993), 45-6.
[29] *Ibid*, 46.
[30] Florence Nightingale said: "It has been said and written scores of times, that every woman makes a good nurse." In: Porter (1997), 378. For Dickens, at least, every *good* woman makes a good nurse.
[31] Quoted in Johnson (1952), 651.
[32] Jacoby (1995), 37.
[33] Markel (1984), 409. This article was excerpted in *Medicine. A Treasury of Art and Literature*. Carmichael and Ratzen, eds. Beaux Arts Editions, New York, 1991, 203-4.
[34] Jones: (1972), 240.
[35] An interesting thought in light of Norman Jacoby's theory that Dickens himself was asthmatic and the autobiographical slant of at least the Mrs Pipchin episode.
[36] Lerner (1997), 156.
[37] Forster (1899), II:23.
[38] For details of Virchow's life and work see e.g.: E.H. Ackerknecht. *Rudolf Virchow. Doctor, Statesman and Anthropologist*. Madison. University of Wisconsin Press, 1953.
[39] In a letter to the *Edinburgh Medical Journal 3*, 1856 Bennett gives the date of his publication as March 19 and Virchow's on August 1, 1845.
[40] Forster (1899), I:172.
[41] Dickens had contact with both Prof Miller and Prof Simpson when Kate suffered a miscarriage in Edinburgh in late 1847. cf: Duncan (1989), 32.
[42] See Forster (1899) I:93.
[43] Schlicke (1999), 628.
[44] Piller (1997), 3.
[45] Fielding (1988), 8 and 15.
[46] Personal communication, April 28, 1999.
[47] Piller (1997), 3.
[48] Personal communication above.
[49] *Harrison's*, 1406.
[50] Weatherall, (1997) 42.
[51] Freedman, (1984), 271.
[52] Forster (1899, II:37-8.

[53] Johnson (1952), 2:605.
[54] Forster (1899), I:7.
[55] See for example "Little Dick" above, or the discussion of Richard Carstone's education in Chapter 13 of *Bleak House.*
[56] Collins (1965), 208.
[57] See Chapter 4. In lay perception, stroke is rare in children, but this is incorrect. Neonates have a stroke incidence equal to that in the elderly (4/1000) and during childhood the rate is still 10/100,000. (Nelson, *The Lancet*, 2002). A brief article in the *Medical Post* (Canada) of March 11, 2003 also reports that stroke is more common in boys than in girls.
[58] This term actually means "hip pain; Jones probably meant "coxitis" or "hip inflammation".
[59] Jones (1972), 240.
[60] Lewis (1992), 1403.
[61] D.F. Cordie (1853). *A Practical Treatise on the Diseases of Children.* Philadelphia: 618-650 [Lewis, 1406].
[62] J. Stewart (1845): *A Practical Treatise on the Diseases of Children*, New York: 291-316 [Lewis, 1406].
[63] Lewis, 1407.
[64] *Ibid.*
[65] Chesney (1993), 818.
[66] Peterson (1993), 818-19.
[67] Pederson (1964), 162.
[68] Callahan (1993), 217.
[69] Nelson (2002), HE01.
[70] Ibid.
[71] Gamble (1996), 25.
[72] Cited in Gamble, (1996), 25.
[73] Gamble (1996), 26.
[74] Cosnett (1999), 1891-2.
[75] Personal communication, January 21, 2000.
[76] Dr David Parker, former Curator of the Dickens Museum, London, in doubting the diagnostic revisions.
[77] "A Killer returns: Scale up the global fight against tuberculosis.' *International Herald Tribune,* March 25, 2003. *The Medical Post* (Canada) of October 13, 2003, brought articles on new TB vaccines currently under development to prevent primary infection (39, 86).

CHAPTER 6: Smallpox

Introduction

Bleak House is by far the most rewarding of Dickens's novels for a reader interested in medical description. Most of the medical references in Dickens's works are found here, ranging from environmental questions to specific diseases and beyond to the inexplicable. The story unfolds in part in a slum area and points an accusing finger at the ruling classes which allow such dreadful conditions to exist cheek-by-jowl with their own opulence. Related to these conditions is the transmission of contagious disease.

Opium use and abuse, domestic violence, infant mortality and illegitimacy play their part, as does the appalling condition of intramural burial grounds. or the reader interested in psychiatry, there are several figures of interest: obsession in the Chancery victims Gridley and Miss Flite; pathological jealousy in the maid, Hortense. In the Smallweed family, the grandmother suffers from senile dementia, having become "weak in her intellect, and [fallen] (for the first time) into a childish state" (*BH*, 264), while the paraplegic grandfather and the granddaughter display signs of sadism.

A relative of the Smallweed family, Krook, is pathologically distrustful and illiterate, or possibly dyslectic.[1] His death by spontaneous combustion is the most spectacular and gruesome scene in the entire book. It brought controversy and scorn as unscientific and utterly impossible; but books on the subject have been published in the twentieth century (see Chapter 10).

Several of the diseases discussed in earlier chapters are found in *Bleak House*, so we focus here on smallpox.

Smallpox as fact and symbol

The longest single medical episode deals with smallpox, which alone, as Michael Gurney, a gastroenterologist, points out

> could so effectively lobby for reform, symbolize a major theme and bring about the transformation of the novel's heroine. Indeed, smallpox is a central unifying force in much of what Dickens is doing in *Bleak House*. It is a testament to his greatness that he is able to accomplish so many artistic and thematic goals while remaining faithful to the properties and symptoms of an actual disease.[2]

In *Bleak House* (1852-3), Dickens "dwelt upon the romantic side of familiar things."[3] Like *Dombey and Son, Bleak House* is a novel of contrasts, but where *Dombey* paired figures or configurations (for example, Mr Dombey/bad father figure vs. Captain Cuttle/good father figure, or the firm of Dombey and Son vs. the Wooden Midshipman), the contrasts in *Bleak House* are oriented to levels of society, the responsibilities among classes and the official institutions and serve to underline their interrelatedness. One basic contrast is the traditional one between the "ugly, unhealthy city" and the "pastoral idyll" of Bleak House and Chesney Wold.[4] Dickens made great use of this theme; but it is only one thread in the mesh of the story. In Chapter 16 Dickens writes:

> What connexion can there be, between the place in Lincolnshire, the house in town, the Mercury in powder, and the whereabouts of Jo the outlaw with the broom, who had that distant ray of light upon him when he swept the churchyard step? What connexion can there have been between many people . . . who, from opposite sides of great gulfs, have, nevertheless, been very curiously brought together (*BH*, 202).

One of the connectors Dickens uses to "curiously bring together" the figures in this novel is disease, specifically, smallpox. It serves as a symbol of the moral contagion in society and also as one link between the city, where it was engendered, and the suburbs, whence it was carried. It links Esther, the illegitimate heroine, and Captain Hawdon, her unknown father. And it creates the hiatus between the repressive childhood Esther experiences at the hands of her "godmother" and the adult awareness needed to overcome the emotional damage to her self-confidence. F.S. Schwarzbach, Professor of English at Washington State University, notes that "Dickens never names the particular fever, but he indicates quite clearly that it is smallpox."[5] This, according to Miriam Bailin, was typical of Victorian fiction in which

> despite an increasingly specific terminology for bodily ailments available to laypersons and medical professionals alike, as well as a decided preference for empirical detail, in fictional representations, the diseases from which the patients suffer remain for the most part unspecified.[6]

The medical historian Charles Rosenberg points out the great familiarity of certain diseases, including smallpox, among the general public. Writing of William Buchan's *Domestic Medicine*,[7] he says

> Buchan felt no need to describe the symptoms of malaria, whooping cough, smallpox or insanity; they were too well known.[8]

Obviously Dickens could also rely on this familiarity and thus did not need to specify which disease he had in mind.

Smallpox and its manifestation

Briefly, to acquaint today's reader with a disease needing no introduction to Victorian readers: Smallpox exists in three forms: *Variola major*, the dangerous, contagious form which was so disfiguring and frequently fatal; *Variola minor* or alastrim, which is much milder; and *Variola vaccinae* or cowpox, a disease of animals which can be transmitted to humans. It is generally uncomplicated and heals without scarring, and, as its Latin name implies, is the source of smallpox vaccine. Though highly contagious, smallpox is less contagious than measles or influenza, and physical contact with persons or contaminated objects is usually required for transmission. The course of the disease consists of an incubation period of about 12 days from the time of exposure to the prodrome, which is characterized by fever, headache and muscle pain abating after 3-4 days. Then the skin eruptions appear, mostly on the face and distal extremities, spreading to the trunk. On the third or fourth day after the rash appears, vesicles develop, and fever returns. Scabs form which usually fall off three weeks after the beginning of illness, leaving the characteristic small scars or deep pits.[9]

Smallpox is now considered eradicated, but it could be counted among the "familiar things" in Dickens's lifetime. There was a major smallpox epidemic from 1837 to 1841 and the disease remained endemic throughout the following decade.[10] A passage in Chapter 22 places the narrative of *Bleak House* squarely in such a period of epidemic events: The law stationer, Mr Snagsby and Inspector Bucket are looking for the crossing-sweeper, Jo, and go into Tom-all-Alone's. They meet a crowd bearing a palanquin and Mr Bucket warns Snagsby to "draw off a bit," since "fever is abroad". Bucket asks his subordinate, Darby, if the nearby houses are the fever houses, to which Darby replies:

> 'all them are', and further that in all, for months and months, the people 'have been down by dozens,' and have been carried out, dead and dying, 'like sheep with the rot.' Bucket observing to Mr Snagsby as they go on again, that he looks a little poorly, Mr Snagsby answers that he feels as if he couldn't breathe the dreadful air (*BH*, 285).

This reflects not only the slum environment, but also Dickens's knowledge of the prevailing medical theory, which hypothesized that disease was caused by miasma - bad air or poisonous gas from rotting organic matter.[11] Fresh air and ventilation were part of every program for urban improvement, from the "Ladies Sanitary Association" to medical councils.

A brief history of vaccination

Smallpox was known and misunderstood for centuries. An undated text by a Taoist scholar, Ko Hung (281-361) refers to smallpox as usually fatal and due to "poisoned air".[12] By the mid-nineteenth century, physicians had realized that the air itself was not necessarily the culprit. Dr Leonard Stuart wrote, for example, in 1837 in *The Lancet,* about influenza:

> We were ignorant of the cause of the disease, but it was evidently directly or indirectly, connected with atmospheric changes; but whether resulting from a physical change in the atmosphere itself, or from the air becoming a vehicle of some noxious matter, was a mystery. All means of prevention were, therefore, unavailable.[13]

This can be applied only to a limited degree to smallpox in Victorian England; of all the infectious scourges afflicting the British public, smallpox was the only one which could, in fact, be prevented. In the Near East, inoculation with active smallpox was practised. Edward Jenner (1749-1823) had discovered in 1796 that the milder cowpox provided adequate protection against smallpox, with almost none of the risks of smallpox inoculation.[14] The first Londoner had been vaccinated in 1798[15] but acceptance of vaccination was not initially wide-spread and was, in fact, slower in Britain than on the continent. In part, resistance was due to vested interests of physicians in the old technique, and in part because the lower classes preferred the familiar inoculation over the new vaccination.[16] A Vaccination Act passed in 1840 provided vaccination as a free medical service, but it was not compulsory in Britain.[17] A problem was caused by administration of the Act by the Poor Law Board, confusing vaccination with a form of parochial relief. Some disadvantages had been reported; vaccination was not always successful and had to be repeated, and there were reports of syphilis transmitted by vaccination. Religious groups protested the use of a vaccine originating in animals. The worst possible argument against vaccination, of course, was that it would eradicate the population-control function of a disease which, after all, reduced mainly that part of the population which was too abundant anyway - namely, the poor.[18]

Compulsory vaccination had not only friends in high medical places, but also opponents in high political places. Sir Robert Peel, Prime Minister when the Act was introduced, declared that

> vaccination, if made compulsory, 'would be so opposite to the mental habits of the British people, and to the freedom of opinion in which they rightly gloried,' that he could be no party to such compulsion.[19]

A mandatory vaccination bill was finally passed in 1853 - the year in which publication of *Bleak House* as a serial was completed and the first bound edition appeared[20] - but the controversy continued, and the bill was submitted for revision in 1866 and again in 1867.

Dickens the editor was not silent on the subject. An article called "Circumlocutional Vaccination" was published in *All the Year Round* in May

1865 setting forth a brief history of vaccination, the current discussion and developments abroad, ending with a plea that Parliament finally heed intelligent arguments and pass the bill. The reason why vaccination was not successful in some cases had meanwhile been discovered: arm-to-arm vaccination had diluted the vaccine to an ineffective level and, in some cases, there was contamination with other infections. The medical world concluded that return to the original source must be attempted. The author of the article (and other Englishmen, no doubt), found it an abomination that the work was continued abroad. The first to act on the conclusion was a physician in Naples, who in 1857 obtained from Queen Victoria a cow infected with cowpox, with which he successfully infected heifers and produced adequate original vaccine to vaccinate thousands of people. His work was known and copied in France - but still not in England. The article concludes:

> Surely England, where the discovery was first made, and which supplied the means of re-establishing the purity of the preservative matter, should not remain behindhand in the race! The frequency with which small-pox has displayed itself in England of late years, the severity not unfrequently attending the cases, and the by no means rare instances of the effects of impure virus, warn us to adopt the very simple remedy within our reach.[21]

Articles in *The Lancet* continued to discuss the Vaccination Bill at length, particularly the attendant politics. As to be expected, when government was involved, there was a great quantity of talk leading - if to anything at all - to the adoption of measures which were not necessarily medically sound. The *Lancet* writer found it, for example, unacceptable that control was to be left largely in the "hands of the guardians of the poor, who have so much else than vaccination to do, and who do that else so badly."[22] The problem of compliance persisted and various means of compulsion were discussed, ranging from a system of certification of successful vaccination as prerequisite to admission to all public service jobs, schools, factories and domestic service, to prosecution for neglect. "A few severe prosecutions," it was argued in the *Lancet* article, "would greatly tend to remove that carelessness which is the explanation of much of the neglect of vaccination."

Transmission of smallpox and its role in the novel

It is entirely possible that "the fever" that Bucket and Mr Snagsby encountered in Tom-All-Alone's was cholera, typhus (usually meant when nineteenth-century laymen said "fever") or typhoid, and not smallpox. Despite the presence of this unnamed "fever," several writers state categorically that Jo got the disease from the graveyard where Nemo was buried. For example, Schwarzbach, who points out that the fog and the mud in the opening words of the novel should be taken quite literally in order not to miss "Dickens's essential message that there are *literal* connections between the mud and fog and Chancery" - writes that "Jo inhales the effluvia given off by the rotting corpse of Nemo, contracts from it smallpox . . ." [23] The argument rests, however, more on establishing yet another link among the various places and people than on evidence in the text, since Nemo died of opium overdose and not smallpox. This interpretation is, however, a fine piece of irony: Esther's father (Nemo) most likely never knew of her existence - though he was still alive the first time she visited Miss Flite, who also lived in Krook's house. He gave her life, biologically, but her only "inheritance" was nearly death.[24]

The incubation period of around 12 days gives Jo time enough after contracting the disease from its source, whatever and wherever it may actually have been, to get to Jenny's - a distance of about 20 miles from London - before becoming obviously ill. The patient with smallpox is infectious from the day *before* the rash breaks out until the lesions have healed and the scabs have fallen off,[25] and this pre-rash, contagious phase is obviously the stage of Jo's disease when he encounters Esther and Charley.

As cited above, smallpox usually requires physical contact for transmission. This knowledge, however, postdates Dickens. For the Victorians, smallpox was the only disease which was considered transmissible by both miasma *and* contact.[26] Dickens might easily have decided on miasma for transmission. It would, in fact, have made his point stronger on the one hand. People could argue that there was little chance of their coming into physical contact with such a figure as Jo, while there was little they could do about air-borne, miasmal diseases. However, physical contact is the one which Dickens selected.[27] Esther reports:

> My little Charley, . . . went quietly up to [Jo] with a chair, and sat him down in it like an old sick nurse (*BH*, 397).

Jo then describes typical symptoms of the prodrome: fever and muscle pain - but there is no mention of a rash. Esther and Charley take the boy home, where Skimpole - who, it must be remembered, was trained in medicine - recommended turning him out: "There's a bad fever about him" (*BH*, 398). Whether Skimpole suspected which fever is not clear - but immaterial, except that Skimpole did know that turning Jo out was to spread the fever further still. This functions to distance the egotistical Skimpole even more from the "model doctor" Allan Woodcourt.[28] The only thing that Skimpole can recommend is that Jo take the medicine Jenny got for him, be kept "moderately warm" and the room "moderately cool" and that a little vinegar be sprinkled around. He later turns the sick boy over to Bucket and we learn in Chapter 46 that Bucket conveyed Jo to a "horsepittle", where he stayed until the worst was over.

Historically interesting in this connection is that the medical community was by no means agreed on the necessity of quarantining patients with infectious diseases within a general hospital. *The Lancet* published part of an 1864 report by Dr J.S. Bristowe and Mr. Timothy Holmes on the hospitals of the UK.[29] These gentlemen saw no reason why typhus cases should not be treated in general wards, as long as the beds were far enough apart and ventilation was adequate; but smallpox patients were to be kept away from the other patients. *The Lancet* author disagreed for reasons of safety to the nursing staff, as well as of lower transmission and mortality rates among patients, for which, like an empirically-minded Victorian, he cited statistics of general hospitals vs. The London Fever Hospital.[30]

Differentiation of smallpox from other possible diseases

Jo is taken away and a search is instituted, which lasts five days. Here, either Jo must be exonerated as the carrier, which, as evident from the working notes for the novel, Dickens did not intend, or Dickens makes a slight error concerning the incubation period: Charley was exposed six days previous to Esther's noticing her malaise and says she had felt the same a day earlier. *Harrison's Principles of Internal Medicine* cites seven days as the extreme lower limit for incubation.[31] Charley's illness progresses rapidly, with high fever and delirium. The disease is indirectly identified by Esther: "I was very sorrowful to think that Charley's pretty looks would change and be disfigured" (*BH*, 403). This is sufficient information for the Victorian reading public to know that Charley has smallpox and not cholera, typhus or typhoid; but to clarify for present readers: Cholera can be ruled out, since the incubation period is only one to three days. There is no disfigurement and recovery is within three to six days in uncomplicated cases. Obviously Charley was seriously ill - and if she had cholera, the chance of death would have been greater than 50%. Also, the full course of the disease in its serious form from onset to death would likely have run within 24 hours.[32]

Cholera can be ruled out on socio-literary grounds as well. Though it was universally feared, it affected only the lower classes, which gave it a negative social connotation beyond its medical importance. It was widely held to be associated with intemperance and immorality,[33] so obviously Esther could not suffer from the disease, though Jo belonged - albeit innocently on his part - to the right milieu.

The second possibility, typhus (a *Rickettsia* infestation transmitted by body lice), begins very much like smallpox. The major and here decisive difference is in the skin eruptions which begin four to seven days after onset of the disease and spread rapidly over the body *except the face.*[34] Moreover, typhus rash does not scar; so typhus can also be ruled out as the diagnosis.

Typhoid is a *Salmonella* infection varying markedly from patient to patient, with an incubation time of 3-60 days (usually about 10). The onset is similar to smallpox and typhus - headache, chills and fever - but the rash develops later, usually during the second week, and appears on the upper abdomen and chest. Mild forms, characterized primarily by fever, may last only a week, but the illness may last eight weeks or more if untreated. Since transmission of *Salmonella typhi* occurs through ingestion of contaminated food, water or milk,[35] it can be ruled out here, since Dickens was careful to include physical contact as the mode in both cases.

By this process of elimination, then, the "diagnosis" of smallpox made above must be correct. That Charley was not scarred is consistent with fact, since she was about thirteen and children usually scarred less than young adults like Esther, who was about twenty-one.

Esther made sure that the rooms were "fresh and airy" (*BH*,403). This had been medical practice from the time of Thomas Sydenham (1624-1672), who published the first clinical description of smallpox.[36] He determined, in Shryock's words, that "smallpox victims . . . need no longer be half-suffocated in closed rooms in addition to their other sufferings."[37] Up to that time "long death-like faints were not uncommon, (since) the stifling system of treating diseases attended with eruption (and especially small-pox) was in vogue."[38]

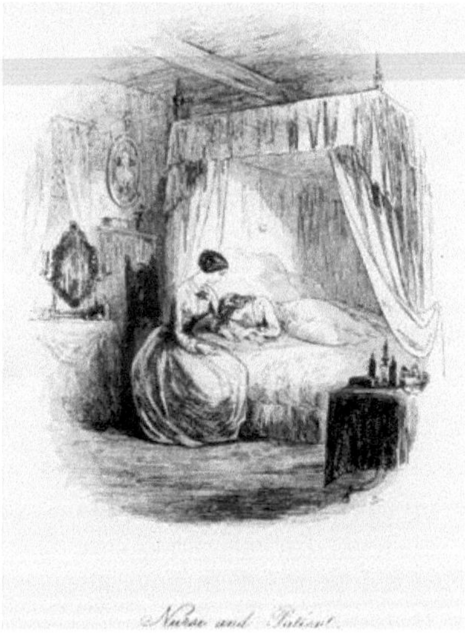

Fig. 8: "Nurse and Patient." *Bleak House*. The Dickens Museum.

Esther nursed Charley in daily close physical contact: ". . . she would be quiet in my arms when she could lie quiet nowhere else" (*BH* 403). Though Esther did "take the air with [her] guardian," she strictly avoided any contact with Ada, and so managed to keep the disease from spreading through Bleak House. Michael Gurney points out that this "self-imposed quarantine . . . makes good sense to us living a century after Pasteur, but it would be strange behavior in a novel whose author believed *only* in miasma as a cause of disease."[39] Thus we have further evidence that Dickens knew of the physical contact element in smallpox contagion.

Dickens's "case reports"

With two people suffering in sequence from the same disease, there are two different descriptions. The first is Esther's objective report of Charley's illness, progress and recovery. The second is the subjective description as Esther herself becomes ill. Since Charley tried to conceal her illness from Esther, we know only of the fever and chills at the end of the prodrome. The prodrome in Esther's case is characterized by confusion and by a feeling of "becoming too large altogether" (*BH*, 404), a bloated feeling commonly associated with high fever and prostration.

Esther becomes temporarily blind; the *Merck Manual of Diagnosis and Therapy* confirms that this is plausible: "The eyes require nursing care if swelling and inflammation are pronounced. It is also possible that the eyes themselves may be affected, which occurs in about 1% of patients."[40] For Dickens and the novel, Esther's blindness serves as the means of directing her vision inward, so that she can finally confront herself as an adult and begin to overcome the emotional damage her rigid upbringing had done to her self-confidence.

Charley had suffered delirium, which Esther reported: "When she was at the worst, and her mind rambled again to the cares of her father's sick-bed . . . [she would] murmur out the wanderings of her mind . . ." (*BH*, 403). Esther's own delirium is reported as confused impressions and dreams. As Esther had reported of Charley, there were lucid intervals in which she "knew perfectly . . . that [she was] in [her] bed" (*BH*, 447) interspersed among visions combining the various phases of her life which she tried to reconcile. She "laboured up colossal staircases" or was part of a "flaming necklace, or ring" from which she wished to be removed.[41]

Dickens himself was interested in the medico-psychological aspects, which is clear from Esther's remark that "It may be that if we knew more of such strange afflictions, we might be the better able to alleviate their intensity" (*BH*, 447). But Philip Collins's warning about misreading Dickens - especially in *Bleak*

House - by translating to "too high a level of abstraction" should be heeded.[42] It is possible to interpret the dreams on the basis of the novel itself, without going off into the great speculation so tempting to the pseudopsychologists. For example, Q.D. Leavis sees Esther's dream as

> representative of the theme of the novel, a nightmare version of what Ada and Richard had debated at the beginning of the novel when they had been inducted into the Chancery world where there is no freewill except in moral decisions. Esther can 'pray to be taken off' and not be a 'part of the dreadful thing,' but it is only by her love and sympathy that she can get off.[43]

Interpretations of Dickens's use of smallpox

Traditional use is obviously made of the trope of the near death/rebirth of the character. Esther, freed from the fear of betraying her mother by her resemblance, can finally free herself of her aunt's disapprobation and realize her potential as an adult woman - including love and marriage. The view that "Dickens indulges Esther's sickness and gives it the amount of space he does because he knows that the romance of sickness and convalescence is good box office"[44] is nonsense. Had Dickens been less careful with details and let Esther alone become dangerously ill - as he did with Rose Maylie in *Oliver Twist*, for example - the jibe might have been accepted. Dickens certainly wrote with an eye to his public and to sales, but the fact that the disease is an easily recognizable one, realistically depicted and yet given literary significance, as well as developmental significance for the character and political significance for society, raises it out of base commercialism.

Joseph Brogunier comments in *The Dickensian* that Esther achieves moral growth as a result of emotional crises and that she is a person of "more humility and self-knowledge" when she "finally accepts the fact that her beauty has been marred by smallpox."[45] This can be accepted to only a limited degree. Since most negative critics of Esther see her "humility" as next-to-nauseating, it is hard to conceive that anyone might call her "more humble" after her illness. Furthermore, moral growth arising from emotional crises is certainly not an Esther-specific novelty, but rather part and parcel of human experience. Esther's situation was not even unique - one of Dickens's major points in the novel - except in the specifics of meeting her mother and being recognized by her after twenty years (one more instance of figures "curiously brought together" by Dickens to weave his story). Literary criticism contains many comments on the fact that Esther is not described anywhere in the book, but there is ample evidence that she was a beautiful young woman. For example, Jenny says after Esther's disfigurement that she could be recognized by her "angel temper, and her pretty shape" (*BH*, 580). The reader knows that Sir Leicester married Lady Dedlock for love and because of her beauty. Since Esther's resemblance to her mother is one important thread in the story, and is quickly recognized by Guppy,[46] it may be assumed that Esther, too, is beautiful, though she is reticent about self-description until after she has been scarred. Even then, for people who have never seen pock-marked individuals, the description is vague. Esther's comment about the danger to Charley's looks was a foreshadowing - and not only for the reader, but for Esther herself. To say that she "finally accepts" the fact of her disfigurement is rather unfair. It must be remembered that the mirrors were taken from her room until she had regained strength. For a pretty, 21-year-old woman in love (though she suppresses this as well as she can), she shows remarkable self-control. It was, of course, not in her nature to complain or rebel; that type of reaction had been trained out of her from infancy.

The outward scarring literally brings to the surface the emotional inner scars of Esther's rigid upbringing. Commentators who complain of Esther's "tedious modesty" underestimate the restraint imposed on an illegitimate child - especially a girl - in the nineteenth century. To begin with, any female child was taught to be self-effacing, obedient and grateful to those who insisted that she be that way. For an illegitimate child, whose existence had "blighted" other lives, the situation was made even worse by a feeling of guilt which was conscientiously instilled. Miss Barbary[47] tells Esther:

> Submission, self-denial, diligent work, are the preparations for a life begun with such a shadow on it. You are different from other children, Esther, because you were not born, like them, in common sinfulness and wrath. (*BH*, 16).[48]

Esther determines to "be industrious, contented, and kind hearted, and to do some good to some one, and win some love to [herself] if [she] could" (*BH*, 16). All the while, however, the guilt and nameless shame which shadow her life make it practically impossible for her to see herself and others' reactions to her objectively. Her steadfast suppression both of her feelings for Allan Woodcourt and any recognition of his feelings for her belong to this constellation. After Esther has been scarred, she interprets Allan's feelings as pity and her typical reaction is that he needs to be consoled. She had not admitted the possibility that he might love and desire her as a woman before he left for India, though both Caddy Jellyby, who brought her the flowers he had left at Miss Flite's, and Ada said the flowers "looked like that sort of thing" (*BH*, 225). Nor can she admit when she meets him later that his emotion could be anything but pity. True to her early resolution to be "content," she accepts Jarndyce's proposal of marriage and it is only through Jarndyce's discernment that she finally "heals" completely. Her passivity belongs to nineteenth-century male-dominated ideals of womanhood and has tended to make criticism of Esther as a character negative. However, Dickens shows considerable insight into the reactions of Esther the child and Esther the prematurely self-controlled young woman who develops out of that child. What would appear to be coy false modesty can clearly be seen as an expression of self-denial vying with the need for proof of self-worth. Esther, as Q.D. Leavis says, "is a very carefully complete study of what a sensitive child is made into in such circumstances as are posited for her."[49]

The end of the book is disturbing to some critics who overlook medical reality and to some extent misread the text. For example, Laura Fasick writes that the

> ambiguity of Woodcourt's final comment about [Esther's] prettiness . . . neither requires nor repays reduction to a single meaning: Whether or not Esther remains scarred is unimportant because Esther's body itself is unimportant. [50]

Fasick sees "good" women in Victorian literature reduced to bodiless souls, whose outward appearance is hidden from the reader's view. But in the case of Esther, as this discussion has attempted to make clear, the outward scars are representational of the inner scars - so it *does* matter whether or not these scars fade. Again, Dickens demonstrates that he is well aware of the details of smallpox. Esther is writing seven years after her marriage, even longer after her illness. Michael Gurney points out that

> [o]ver the first several months following an infection, the scars become hyperpigmented, further accentuating their presence. Fortunately, this pigmentation often faded over the years and scars lost their depth, occasionally to the point of complete disappearance.[51]

The novel makes clear that Esther, having regained her physical health, has also attained a new emotional health. She has not been permanently altered in looks, and she was not even temporarily altered in her charity, kindness and sense of duty, which are Dickens's recommendation for the treatment of the ills of society.

While Dickens's recommendation was able to effect changes, even he was aware that there were some matters in which centralization of effort was essential if the evils were to be eradicated. The issues covered now by the term "public health" are certainly among these, and we now turn our attention to a complicated and necessarily selective chapter on public health in the Victorian England of Dickens's lifetime.

[1] This question was addressed by the pediatrician Norman Jacoby in the *Dickensian*, 91 (1995):102-107, but his verdict of "dyslexic" was criticized by at least one teacher of dyslexic children, K.E. Cole of King's College. *The Dickensian*, 91 (1995):209-210.

[2] Gurney (1990), 90.

[3] Preface to the book version of the novel, August 1853.

[4] This trope was attacked in Charles Kingsley's *Yeast* (1848), who rejected the idea that dirt and disease existed only in industrial towns and that life in the country was healthy.

[5] Schwarzbach (1990), 103, Note 11.

[6] Bailin (1994), 7.

[7] William Buchan (1729), 1805. See also Chapter 8 below.

[8] Rosenberg (1983), 27. Rosenberg also points out that Buchan's book was modelled on S.A. Tissot's *Avis au peuple sur la santé* (1761), so, in addition to epilepsy, we can postulate another indirect connection between Tissot and Dickens.

[9] *Harrison's,* 799.

[10] Gurney (1990), 81.

[11] Schwarzbach (1990) comments that raw sewage etc. "ends in the Thames and then oozes downstream to the Essex marshes. There it rots and festers, soon producing infectious effluvia that are blown by the raw East Wind back over the city" (Schwarzbach, 95). This is another point known to Victorians perhaps missed by modern readers, who wonder why the wind was in the east when Jarndyce was upset about anything.

[12] Seiffert and Du Dscheng-Hsing (1937), 26.

[13] *The Lancet,* January 30, 1837:677.

[14] Shryock (1948), 70.

[15] Gurney (1990), 83.

[16] Baldwin (1999), 253.

[17] Unlike in Bavaria, Scandinavia and Russia where it became compulsory as early as 1816. (Gurney (1990), 81).

[18] One is reminded of Scrooge's comment that "if [the poor] be like to die, they had better do it and reduce the surplus population" in the *Christmas Carol*, 10 years before *Bleak House*. Dickens had no need to repeat that here, since his readers would have been well aware of the argument.

[19] Quoted in *The Lancet*, March 9, 1867:304.

[20] This is not purely coincidence; see Anthony Trollope, *The Warden* (1855) and his comments on "Mr Sentiment."

[21] *AYR* 13:376-7. The author of this article is - as usual in *AYR* - unidentified..

[22] Article dated Saturday, May 11, 1867, 570.

[23] Schwarzbach (1990), 96; original emphasis.

[24] Lyn Pykett (2002) includes in the link between Nemo and Jo "the spreading of the smallpox, which kills one character and, for a time, disfigures another" (Pykett, 134). This is incorrect, since none of the characters in *BH* dies of smallpox.

[25] *Harrison's,* 799; my emphasis.

[26] They were not entirely mistaken; airborne dissemination has been shown to occur. *Harrison's*, 799.

[27] It is, as we know now, also the more medically correct. Whether Dickens knew this, or surmised as much, is a question we cannot answer.

[28] One of Dickens's most exasperated statements can be found in this passage, namely when he speaks through Jarndyce:

"Is it not a horrible reflection. . .that if this wretched creature were a convicted prisoner, his hospital would be wide open to him, and he would be as well taken care of as any sick boy in the kingdom?" (398).

[29] *The Lancet,* February 11, 1865.
[30] *AYR* contained an article entitled "Growth of a Hospital" soliciting funds on behalf of the London Fever Hospital and its work (5:475).
[31] *Harrison's,* 799.
[32] Gurney (1990), 89.
[33] Ibid, 90.
[34] *Merck Manual*, (1977), 67-8.; [*Merck*] my emphasis.
[35] *Harrison's*, 641-2.
[36] Castiglioni (1975), 546-7.
[37] Shryock (1948), 21.
[38] This was also described in an article entitled "Medical Nuts to Crack", *All the Year Round,* 5, 358-60; author unidentified. The story cited was that of an infant girl who had small-pox, was kept in a closed room and "died", but revived when the room was aired.
[39] Gurney (1990), 82, my emphasis.
[40] *Merck*, 85.
[41] Being part of something surreal and wanting to be released occurs again in Pip's dream in *Great Expectations* after Magwitch's death (*GE*, 444). The imagery there is more masculine, the medical state is different, but the dreams are comparable.
[42] Collins in: Almaric (1973), 163.
[43] Leavis (1994 reprint), 216.
[44] Carter, in Cox (1984), 143.
[45] Brogunier (1965), 60.
[46] though ostensibly not by her almost-uncle Boythorn, who had been engaged to "Miss Barbary," or Jarndyce, who had known Lady Dedlock before her marriage.
[47] A speaking name to ensure the reader's awareness that Dickens disapproves her behaviour.
[48] This attitude, and the religious objections to using vaccines from animals, may explain why Esther had not been vaccinated.
[49] Leavis (1994 reprint), 212.
[50] Fasick (1996), 142.
[51] Gurney (1990), 86.

CHAPTER 7: Public Health

Introduction

A chapter on public health is indispensable to any study broadly dealing with nineteenth-century medicine. Almost limitless historical information is available, since the Victorian Age marks the beginning of public health as it is known today. New concepts of sanitation and housing were the one positive effect of the panic wrought by epidemic disease. The importance of cholera in the initiation of public health measures in the nineteenth century can hardly be overestimated. And Dickens's importance was recorded in a pamphlet published in 1853:

> There have been at work among us three great social agencies: the London City Mission, the novels of Mr Dickens, and the cholera.[1]

In this chapter I examine some of the many aspects of public health in Victorian England of which Dickens made pointed and topical use in his fiction. Dickens's concern with matters of public health is even more directly addressed in articles published in his weekly journals and in his speeches (see Appendix 4). Personal acquaintance and friendship with some of the leading figures in the sanitation reform movement, like Sir Edwin Chadwick and Dr Thomas Southwood Smith, gave Dickens ready access to information on developments as well as on obstacles arising in the passing of legislation. As almoner to Angela Burdett-Coutts, he also helped to initiate direct specific improvements in housing and sanitation for at least some of London's population.

Although some critics class Dickens among the great reformers of the Victorian age, he was not a reformer in the sense of, for example, Chadwick. He did not *create* the impetus to reform, nor did he preach any definite program by which reform was to be carried out. As Virginia Berridge points out "The sanitary movement was very much a matter of effective propaganda and the creation of a responsive climate of opinion."[2] Dickens's function was to call attention to the problem, making the middle and upper classes aware of the conditions under which much of the population lived and of their obligation to assist in changing those conditions.[3] In his skepticism and distrust of governmental activities, Dickens, like Dr Buchan before him, looked "to individual, not collective remedies for health problems which seemed to be social and potentially remediable."[4]

The present discussion is confined to certain specific topics in their Victorian setting: feeding and care of motherless children, sanitation and housing, free sale of poisons, metropolitan burial grounds, bodysnatching and the Anatomy Law, and substance abuse. Examples of Dickens's fictional use of these subjects are given, along with both historical information and Dickens-contemporary witness in medical journals and the lay press, including in a very few instances Dickens's journals, to underline the topicality of Dickens's writings. Hospitals, which were not public institutions for the most part, play only a minor role in Dickens's fiction and are therefore not included here, but reference to his speeches and articles for the benefit of particular hospitals is found in the appendix.

One of the major problems in the Victorian Age, and one particularly close to Dickens's heart, involved poor or orphaned children. As society's weakest link, they required special consideration of their physical, emotional and medical needs. The sociomedical problem of how to raise a motherless child became a public health problem in its impact on infant mortality rates and in its later impact due to the survivors' retarded development and susceptibility to illness.

The feeding of infants

One problem emergent in the Industrial Revolution - and still current - is care for the children of working mothers. Dickens addressed this obliquely in his second Christmas Story *The Chimes* written in Genoa in 1844. He had addressed the true Christmas (= Christian, in his definition) spirit in the first of his Christmas books in 1843. In his second, he

> was out to strike the heaviest blow in his power on behalf of the poor and oppressed of early Victorian England . . . .[5]

In *The Chimes*, Sir Joseph Bowley, MP, prides himself on being the "Poor Man's Friend." Michael Slater's notes on the text point out that the figure was undoubtedly based on the Whig ex-Chancellor Lord Brougham, a self-proclaimed philanthropist. In 1844, when the Factory Bill was introduced to limit work to 10 hours per day, supporters argued, among other things, that

> the children of women factory-workers suffered from malnutrition, as their mothers had no leisure to feed them. Brougham observed that peeresses and MPs' wives were also often prevented 'by their various avocations' from suckling *their* children, but he 'had never heard that any mischief resulted from the practice.'

This speech occasioned a bitter attack by Douglas Jerrold in *Punch* (April 6, 1844) entitled "Lord Brougham on Wet-Nurses".[6]

An essential feature of society for various reasons until the late nineteenth century, wet-nurses were not generally available to poor people, who were more apt to be suppliers than consumers. Dickens was well-acquainted with the matter: the second chapter of *Dombey and Son,* entitled "In which Provision is made for an emergency that will sometimes arise in the best-regulated Families", details the problem of providing sustenance for a motherless neonate. In Western societies of the twenty-first century, there is hardly a problem of maternal death in childbed, or of death of full-term neonates. For the Victorians, however, both were common and each was coupled with its own special problems. Chapter 2 of *Dombey* can, of course, be read strictly in its relation to the entire novel. It introduces Mrs Chick, Miss Tox and the Toodle family. It provides several of the many contrasts in the work: family life à la Toodle versus family life à la Dombey; a frank, open workman producing numerous, healthy sons without losing his wife, versus a repressed, egocentric businessman producing only two children, losing his wife at the birth of his obsessively-awaited són, who also dies young.[7] It also contrasts the hierarchy among the servants above and below stairs, as well as the closed society of a defined group and the larger society of which they are part. It provides an introduction to Paul Dombey, Sr in his dealings with his "inferiors" and also his dreams and self-delusions.

But at a different level, as the heading indicates, the chapter addresses the age-old problem of how to feed a motherless infant. Historically, wet-nursing has been the preferred method whenever possible. In other cases, the ancient Greeks and Romans used so-called "gutti" - instruments made of clay or glass, which could be emptied drop-wise into the infant's mouth. Starting in the thirteenth century, cow's horns were used. These were replaced by ceramic or wood bottles in the fifteenth to seventeenth centuries. Heinrich von Louffenburg (ca. 1458) wrote the first paediatric text depicting a feeding bottle of a design still in use today.[8] Metal bottles of tin or silver with a metal suction cap covered with leather or fabric were introduced in the early nineteenth century.[9]

Apparently, none of these possibilities occurs to anyone in the Dombey household - except Mr Chick, who reaps scorn from his wife for his trouble. First, he confuses dry nurse and wet nurse; then he makes what his wife considers a totally absurd suggestion:

> 'It would have occurred to most men,' said Mrs Chick, 'that poor dear Fanny being no more . . . it becomes necessary to provide a Nurse.'
>
> 'Oh! Ah!' said Mr Chick. 'Toor-rul - such is life, I mean. I hope you are suited, my dear.'
>
> 'Indeed I am not,' said Mrs Chick, 'nor likely to be, so far as I can see. Meanwhile, of course, the child is -'
>
> 'Going to the the very Deuce,' said Mr Chick, thoughtfully, 'to be sure.'
>
> Admonished, however, that he had committed himself . . . and thinking to atone for his misconduct by a bright suggestion, he added:
>
> 'Couldn't something temporary be done with a teapot?'(*DS*, 62/3).

This is an amusing incident of male helplessness camouflaged by facetiousness in confronting a basically female problem. But was it merely Dickens's humour, or is there an autobiographical slant? Dickens's first child, Charlie, was about nine when *Dombey* began publication. A letter from Dickens's sister-in-law Mary Hogarth to her cousin Mary Scott shortly after Charlie's birth reports that

> Kate, . . . I am sorry indeed to say has not gone on so well as her first week made us hope she would. . . . it was discovered she was not able to nurse her Baby, so she was obliged . . . to give him up to a stranger. . . . She has got a very nice Nurse for him . . .[10]

Dickens seems to have made no direct mention of this in his correspondence. But perhaps the young Dickens - less than a month before his twenty-fifth birthday – (or his father?) made the remark which got Mr Chick in trouble with his wife.

The idea of a teapot was not so absurd. Feeding vessels have been found on Cyprus dating from about 400 BC which are not unlike a teapot. And Dr Hugh Smith designed a "bubby pot" for feeding infants, which he described in the third edition of his popular book: *Letters to married women* (1774) as "not unlike a coffee pot." There was also a device of similar design used for force-feeding mental patients who refused nourishment. If he was unaware of the other feeding vessels, perhaps Dickens knew of this from his friend Dr John Conolly, who headed a large hospital for the insane at Hanwell.

Recruitment of wet-nurses

Curiously, it is the unmarried Miss Tox who finds the solution to the problem. Several candidates have been interviewed for the job and rejected, when Miss Tox appears with the Toodle family.

> 'My dear Louisa,' said Miss Tox, 'knowing your great anxiety, ... I posted off myself to the Queen Charlotte's Royal Married Females,[11] . . . and put the question, Was there anybody there that they thought would suit? No, they said there was not. .... But . . . one of the Royal Married Females, hearing the inquiry, reminded the matron of another who . . . would in all likelihood be most satisfactory. The moment I heard this, and had it corroborated by the matron - excellent references and unimpeachable character - I got the address, my dear, and posted off again' (*DS*, 15/6).

Who performed this service for the Dickens family is not found in available records. But it is obvious that Dickens knew about the hospital, a major source of wet-nurses in London.[12] He also apparently knew that the wet nurse should be "amiable, sober, civil and her home clean" and that she should "have had two or three children of her own."[13] In ancient times, it would even have been stipulated that, since she was to nurse a male child, her last child should have been male, since the milk supposedly had a different quality if the infant was male or female. Brunettes were thought to produce the most breast milk, while redheads were viewed as the poorest choice for a wet-nurse.[14]

Mr Dombey's first reaction to the "two rosiest" of the Toodle family is that they look healthy. "But to think of their some day claiming a sort of relationship to Paul!" (*DS*, 17). Portrayed throughout as proud and selfish, he gives no thought to Polly or to her youngest, unweaned child, who is only six weeks old. Polly is found acceptable, separated from her family and her identity - Mr Dombey insisting on calling her Richards - and begins her new job, leaving her unmarried sister, Jemima, to care for her children. Miss Tox and Mrs Chick hold out special treatment as a consolation for Polly's being separated from her family:

> 'As to living, Richards, you know, . . . anything you take a fancy to, I'm sure will be as readily provided as if you were a Lady' (*DS*, 22).

Lionel Rose points out that the "higher classes took these women under their roofs to queen it among the servants."[15] This cannot be claimed of "Richards," and she was certainly viewed askance by Susan Nipper, who sharply reminded her that Miss Floy was "a permanency and Master Paul a temporary" (*DS*, 27). Polly is with the family "six months or so" (*DS*, 64) when she is won over by Susan Nipper to the indiscretion of visiting her family in Staggs's Gardens, leading to her dismissal. How much longer she would have been employed is a moot point here; but Chapter 6 is entitled "Paul's Second Deprivation."

Chapter 5, "Paul's Progress and Christening" opens with the words: "Little Paul, suffering no contamination from the blood of the Toodles, grew stouter and stronger every day." This sounds strange now, but it was very familiar to Victorian readers and, indeed, goes back to the ancients. Both the church and the medical profession were convinced that inherited traits could be passed from a woman via breast-milk to the suckling infant. Even more horrible to contemplate was the result of drinking the milk of an animal. A 14th century Tuscan text warns:

> Be sure that the wet nurse has plenty of milk, because if she lacks it she may give the baby the milk of a goat . . . or some other animal, because the child . . . nourished on animal milk does not have perfect wits like one fed on women's milk, but always looks stupid and vacant and not right in the head.[16]

The discussion continued well after publication of *Dombey*. For example, *The Lancet* of January 29, 1859 carried an article on page 113 about recruiting wet-nurses from "fallen women." One of those complaining of the animosity against the plan and writing in support of the attempt was William Acton, whose famous book *Prostitution Considered in its Moral, Social, and Sanitary Aspects in London and other Large Cities and Garrison Towns with Proposals for the Control and Prevention of its Attendant Evils* had been published two years earlier. In a letter to the *The Lancet* on February 12, 1859, Acton points out that the demand for wet-nurses has always been greater than the supply. He is very careful to stress that

> it is not street-walkers nor professional prostitutes we are speaking of. We are speaking of the young house-maid or pretty parlour-maid in the same street in which the sickly lady has given birth to a sickly child, to whom healthy milk is life, and anything else death.

It is noted that Acton does not say what should happen with the illegitimate baby, which frequently had to be given up and "raised by hand," which was associated with a high mortality rate.

The doctor, says Acton, must ascertain that the young woman is healthy to prevent a woman of "undesirable character" from passing an undetected syphilis to the child, but contrary to popular prejudice, he denies any moral effect at all:

> As to any permanent moral effect, I need only state the fear to calm it. . . With what omniscient power should the previous lives, nay the thoughts and feelings, of all nurses - ay, and mothers - be scrutinized, if this be true! And how many infants, had we this power, would be condemned to the pap-bottle, indigestion and the grave!

Acton would probably not have approved of Polly Toodle. He writes:

> You cannot get married women, or, if you do, they are of a kind that make the anxious doctor long after the unmarried. A married woman who voluntarily leaves her own child for money may not be much better than the girl accidentally seduced, who nurses another's child for bread.

Acton paraphrases here a text published about 1584:

> Ill, will the bus'ness by that nurse be done,
> Who for another's child neglects her own.[17]

"Raising by hand"

Wet-nurses were not always available, and not everyone knew about Smith's "bubby pot". What happened to motherless children in such cases? There was no baby formula as we know it today, and the "hand-rearing of babies was necessarily attended by malnutrition and enteric disorders under even the most well-intentioned regime."[18]. In hospitals, the solution to the problem was frequently a long-tubed feeding bottle. This device "allowed the busy [hospital] nurse to leave the infant, while the feed was siphoned automatically from the bottle, which rested on a ledge." Of course, the flow could be impeded, or the bottle empty, or the child too weak to reach the tube, in which case the device was "popular but quite lethal." [19]

As illegitimate, unwanted children, we can only speculate on the way in which Esther Summerson (*BH*) and Arthur Clennam (*LD)* were fed as infants. The parish doctor recommended giving the new-born Oliver Twist "a little gruel" if he cried; what happened later is not recorded. Pip (*GE*) is constantly reminded that his sister had "brought him up by hand" – making it rather a wonder that the child had survived – but we don't know whether Miss Barbary and Mrs Clennam felt that their "Christian" duty required hiring a wet nurse. It is perhaps more likely that they would not consciously have hoped for, but at least have accepted the child's early death as "God's will" and put on a hypocritical face of "sorrow."

Baby Farms

There were several means of disposing of an orphaned or unwanted baby. One example of practical charity in this regard was set by Thomas Coram, who funded the London Foundling Hospital in 1739. The name is rather misleading, since the hospital was intended for the infants of "innocent, deceived girls" who were interviewed to make sure they fulfilled this criterion. In order to be allowed to leave the child there, the child had to be the first born and preference was given to cases in which some promise of marriage had been made to the mother, or some other form of deception practised upon her. She must never have lived with the child's father. The object of these restrictions is as much to effect the restoration of the mother to society, as to provide for her child.[20] An important secondary role is played in *Little Dorrit* by Tattycoram, whose name was really Harriet Coram and whose "family" name was taken from the Foundling Hospital in Coram Fields. The child's treatment by the Meagles's, while well-intentioned, served only to alienate her.[21] It cannot be ruled out that this misguided behaviour was related to the child's illegitimacy.

Another possibility was to "farm" the child. Sometimes, these "farms" were paid for by the parish. This is the form which Dickens used for the orphaned Oliver Twist, who was placed under the "care" of Mrs Mann.

> … the parish authorities magnanimously and humanely resolved, that Oliver should be "farmed" or, in other words, that he should be despatched to a branch-workhouse some three miles off, where twenty or thirty other juvenile offenders against the poor-laws rolled about the floor all day, without the inconvenience of too

much food or too much clothing, under the parental superintendence of an elderly female (*OT*, 3-4).

One real-life "farm" appears nearly twenty years later in a major Dickens novel, namely in *Bleak House* (1851-53). The law stationer, Mr Snagsby, has a housemaid, Guster, who had been farmed "to an amiable benefactor of his species resident at Tooting." More is said of this in connection with Guster in Chapter 3. It is noted here that the "amiable benefactor" is – as might be expected in light of Dickens's sympathy with poor and abused children - bitter irony.

In the *BMJ* of June 18, 1870, an article appeared complaining that, while the *Journal* had attacked the practice of baby farming in 1868, nothing had changed. There was still

> the usual scenery of a baby-farm – the half-dozen children lying dirty and emaciated, huddled on a sofa, quiet and asleep, drugged and half-starved; nursing bottles with sour milk, and a weak mixture of cornflour.

To say this hadn't changed since 1868 is putting it mildly; when this text is compared with the quotation from *Oliver Twist*, cited above, it is seen that nothing had changed during the previous 30 years, either.

Sanitation/Housing

Even when the child was not orphaned and not farmed out due to poverty, the conditions under which it – and its family – lived were frequently appalling. This was one of the issues against which Dickens protested most frequently and most vociferously.

It can be argued that the ancient Romans had implemented many if not most of the sanitation measures. But with the fall of the Roman Empire, the systems were allowed to go to rack and ruin. Rediscovery of the principles was mandated by the problems of the Industrial Age, since industrialization and the massing of population in industrial centres brought a devastating increase in mortality. The cities simply could not provide adequate housing, waste management and potable water to the burgeoning population. The physician and civil servant, William Farr (1897-1883) considered the higher rate of urban over rural mortality to be due more to a lack of sanitation than to poverty itself. But Edwin Chadwick (1800-1890) a civil servant and utilitarian who had drafted the New Poor Law of 1834, saw the direct connection between poverty and disease. His initial interest was caught by the costs involved in providing relief for families left destitute when the bread-winner died of what he considered preventable disease. Indeed, public health reform in Britain "resulted from a mixture of philanthropic relief, political expediency and, most of all, from utilitarian principles of political economy."[22]

In 1837 Chadwick called on Neil Arnott (1788-1844), James Kaye-Shuttleworth (1804-1871) and Dr Thomas Southwood Smith (1788-1861) to investigate conditions in the London districts with the highest mortality rates. Their work was subsequently expanded to include other parts of Great Britain and culminated in the "Report on the Sanitary Conditions of the Labouring Population of Great Britain" in 1842. Partly as a result of this work, Southwood Smith and a group of colleagues formed the Metropolitan Health of Towns Association in 1844. The Honorary Secretary of the group was a civil engineer, Henry Austin, who also worked closely with Edwin Chadwick. Austin, whom Dickens had known since youth,[23] was married to Dickens's younger sister, Laetitia, a connection of mutual benefit, since Austin could rely on Dickens to espouse the cause of sanitation reform, and Dickens could rely on Austin for inside information on topics under discussion by the Association. Dickens himself became a member of the Association, but not until 1848, shortly before the Health of Towns Bill was passed, bringing the Association's work to a close.

On February 6, 1850, Dickens spoke at the first public meeting of the Metropolitan Sanitary Association, an organization formed because London had been excluded from the provisions of the Public Health Act in 1847 – "most absurdly and monstrously" in Dickens's words.[24] He also spoke at the first anniversary banquet of the Association on May 10, 1851, saying that

> no-one can estimate the amount of mischief which is grown in dirt; that no-one can say, here it stops, or there it stops...that if you once have a vigorous pestilence raging furiously in Saint Giles's, no mortal list of Lady Patronesses can keep it out of Almacks. . . . [A]ll the information I have ... been able to acquire through any of my senses, has strengthened me in the conviction that Searching Sanitary Reform must precede all other social remedies, and that even Education and Religion can do nothing where they are most needed, until the way is paved for their ministrations by Cleanliness and Decency.[25]

Although Dickens was strongly opposed to the Poor Law drafted by Chadwick as being too harsh and unfair to the underprivileged, he warmly supported Chadwick's work for improvement in sanitation. There is mention of Chadwick in several articles in the journals, and the penultimate section of *American Notes for General Circulation* (1842) closes with the words:

> There is no local Legislature in America which may not study Mr Chadwick's excellent Report upon the Sanitary Condition of our Labouring Classes, with immense advantage.

Dr Southwood Smith and Dickens became personal friends and the two collaborated on a variety of projects, including some financed by Angela Burdett-Coutts.

Dickens's interest in sanitation and housing is evident as early as the *Sketches by Boz* (1835). His descriptions of certain parts of London were likely a revelation for many of his readers who had never ventured far outside their own quarters. "Seven Dials" for example, has

> streets of dirty, straggling houses, with now and then an unexpected court composed of buildings as ill-proportioned and deformed as the half-naked children that wallow in the kennels (*SB*, 73).

In Drury Lane, there are

> "wretched houses with broken windows patched with rags and paper: every room let out to a different family, and in many instances to two or even three -..." (*SB*, "Gin-Shops", 183).

In the Preface to the first Cheap Edition of *Martin Chuzzlewit*, published in November 1849 and dedicated to Angela Burdett-Coutts, Dickens wrote "I hope I have taken every available opportunity of showing the want of sanitary improvements in the neglected dwellings of the poor."[26] Certainly examples of such writings are easily identified; one need only think of the descriptions in *Oliver Twist* (1837-39) of Fagin's den or Jacob's Island (the existence of which was denied by Sir Peter Laurie[27]); or Good Mrs Brown's dwelling in *Dombey & Son* (Chapter 6; 1846-48). Perhaps the most pointed description is that of the brickmaker's dwelling in *Bleak House* (Chapter 8; 1851-53), which presents opposing interpretations of what is seen. Mrs Pardiggle talks "with much volubility about the untidy habits of the people" while Esther doubts that "the best of us could have been tidy in such a place." Not only does Dickens describe the area as a "cluster of wretched hovels in a brickfield, with pigsties close to the broken windows, and miserable little gardens before the doors, growing nothing but stagnant pools", he also emphasises the lack of clean water and relates it to the high infant mortality of the time:

> "Look at the water. Smell it! That's wot we drinks. How do you like it, and what do you think of gin, instead? An't my place dirty? Yes, it is dirty – it's nat'rally dirty, and it's nat'rally onwholesome; and we've had five dirty and onwholesome children, as is all dead infants, and so much the better for them, and for us besides" (*BH*, 98).

That much could – and should – be done by Government, individuals and associations to correct the miserable conditions under which a considerable portion of the population lived was recognized, discussed, written about and finally acted upon. Much of the groundwork was laid by the Metropolitan Sanitary Association and the Board of Health under Sir Edwin Chadwick, as mentioned above. *The Lancet* set up its own Analytical Sanitary Commission, which, in addition to its other activities, investigated pollution of the Thames in 1851. Part of this report appears to have had some influence on Dickens's writing of the passage from *BH* cited above:

> ...the water of the poor is nearly always exposed to noxious gases and agencies which arise from privies and the slow decomposition of the refuse in their yards, and also from their close, offensive and impure dwellings...

But what was to be done about these "close, offensive and impure dwellings?" Dickens was only one of many who pondered the question and raised it in public over and over again. One project in which Dickens was personally involved was financed by Angela Burdett Coutts. According to K.J. Fielding, Miss Coutts evidently turned her attention to housing in 1852, and

> in taking an active interest in the great task of improving the homes of the poor in London, she began to advance, with Dickens's help, beyond a narrow scope of merely private charity to become one of the leading practical philanthropists and pioneers in social work of the century.[28]

Dickens suggested consulting his friend, Dr Southwood Smith, who, as a member of the General Board of Health, was well acquainted with all the worst districts in London. Probably the decision to buy land in Bethnal Green was based on Southwood Smith's recommendation. The area was undrained and overshadowed by a huge dustheap. Miss Coutts hired a well-known architect, Philip Hardwick, to survey the land, and Dickens recommended that before she approved any plans, she again consult his brother-in-law, Henry Austin, and Southwood Smith. For some reason, apparently related to moving the dustheap, work was not started until 1859 and the block of flats was opened sometime in 1862. These were known as Columbia Buildings, or Columbia Square, and an article about them appeared in *AYR* on June 7, 1862 "Hail Columbia – Square!" Fielding is of the opinion that the article was "probably by W.H. Wills" – no author is cited in Ella Ann Oppenlander's index of articles.[29] The article evokes *D&S*, Chapter 20 with its description of the things Mr Dombey sees from his carriage window, and even more Chapter 47: "Oh for a good spirit who would take the house-tops off, with a more potent and benignant hand than the lame demon in the tale..." In the article,

> many travellers starting on a leisure-trip have an Asmodeus glimpse of courts and alleys, and houses and rooms, which they would otherwise never see ... It will be great comfort to know that such misery may be alleviated . . . and that the frightful

conditions in which the poor exist is not an inevitable and irremediable evil, but, on the contrary, one to which it is perfectly simple and easy to apply a remedy, if we will but exert ourselves in the right direction.[30]

The design of the complex is briefly described – well-ventilated, with a kitchen in each flat, communal laundry provided with a centrifuge. And all of this earns money – 3%, which is not considered sufficient to interest a speculator, but "solid and reliable". This self-supporting aspect is the "surest foundation" for homes for the poor, in which the "barest, commonest decency, and the preservation of health" are the two most important features.

In January 1854, *Household Words* carried an article by Henry Morley entitled "Your Very Good Health", which summarized certain "Results of Sanitary Improvement" which had "lately been published in a little tract by that indefatigable and useful sanitary reformer, Dr Southwood Smith". The tract describes in particular the effect which improved sanitation had on the prevention of cholera, comparing the results of mortality due to unsanitary conditions in various years. Morley concludes:

> The 23000 Londoners, fewer or more, who in this year 1854, are otherwise to die through the want of a complete sanitary system, had better bestir themselves and look after reforms. The difficulty is to know, . . . which of us are to be enlisted in the army of dead men claimed yearly by King Dirt.[31]

One of the most virulent "recruiting stations" for the "army of dead men" was to be found in the graveyards of the city. This was the subject of extra legislation and also addressed by Dickens. In the following we turn our attention to related matters, that is, to the condition of graves and grave-yards, and further to the desecration of graves by bodysnatchers prior to the passing of the Anatomy Act in 1832.

Metropolitan Burials

Burial in churches

The dangers inherent in intramural sepulture had long since been recognized and addressed; this was not a "new discovery" by nineteenth-century medicine or sanitary engineers. One example of a treatise on the subject written more than a century before Dickens began his career dates from 1721. Written by A. Bettesworth of Sandwich, it bears the long title: *Seasonable Considerations on the Indecent and Dangerous Custom of Burying in Churches and Church-Yards with remarkable Observations Historical and Philosophical Proving that the Custom is not only Contrary to the Practice of the Antients,*[sic] *but Fatal, in Case of Infection*. Bettesworth reports that in Rome, only the emperor and vestal virgins could be buried within the city walls. Theodosius I (AD 346?-395), who first made Christianity the official religion of the Roman Empire, decreed that the churches of the apostles and martyrs were not designed as burial places of the dead, and continued the ban.

In England, Cuthred, 13th King of the West Saxons (†756) was the first to permit burial within city walls, while Cuthbert, the 10th Archbishop of Canterbury (from 740-760), first obtained a privilege from the Pope to use churchyards for interment. In Bettesworth's opinion, the motivation behind burying in or near churches was threefold: Pride and Ambition; Superstition and Error; and Gain and Lucre. As an example of the first he cites Constantin, who could not be buried in a church, but in order to be as close as possible, was "buried in the Porch of the great Church at Constantinople, which he had most magnificently built, Anno 337, to the Honour of the Twelve Apostles, not excluding his own."[32] With respect to superstition, Bettesworth reports that the grave nearest the altar was esteemed the most "vertuous" [*sic*], and consequently to be purchased at any price. This leads him to point out that the burial of the dead in or near the church was a source of gain and lucre for the church, or at least for the sexton and priest.

Bettesworth's objection to the practice is that

> It is an undoubted Truth, that the Corruption of Dead Bodies interred in Churches may be communicated to the Living; and that many dangerous and fatal Distempers may be received from the Effluvia of the Dead by secret communication, although the Stench be not perceived by the Nostrils. [33]

He goes on to point out that the cause of death plays a role in whether the effluvia are noxious or not, and that physicians advise not burying anyone in churches in times of pestilence. They also recommend "smoking the churches" before the congregation assembles. Bettesworth speculates from this that the danger of contagion must be greater in protestant churches, since "Popish Churches . . . are at all times fumigated by Incense, and Lamps continually burning, which may in some Degree, destroy the Vapours."[34]

Whether Dickens mentions anything unpleasant or noxious in connection with the church depends on the atmosphere he wishes to create in the particular novel.[35] The first description of the interior of an old church is found in Chapter 53 of *The Old Curiosity Shop.* Nell and her grandfather have found refuge with the schoolmaster and Nell has been given the job of showing the church to visitors. Predominant in the description of the church are dust and decay, but certainly without any noxious influences. Dickens is setting the scene for the child's death and burial in the church. Despite all manner of hardships and trials, there has been nothing to sully the pure image of Little Nell, and the description of dusty, but not defiled, tombs among which Nell and her grandfather will themselves lie, maintains that end.

Interior scenes in churches do not appear again in Dickens's novels until *Dombey and Son,* and here is mention of "a strange, unusual, uncomfortable smell" in the church when Paul is christened (Chapter 5). Although the baptism must wait until a wedding is over, there is nothing welcoming about the church, even in the celebrations of life. It is cold, damp, grim and filled with "cadaverous light". Here, Dickens begins preparing the reader for Paul's death. He – like his mother – is buried in the church.

The second church to be mentioned in *Dombey* is "a mouldy old church in a yard, hemmed in by a labyrinth of back streets and courts, with a little burying-ground round it." Since this is the scene of Florence Dombey's marriage to Walter Gay, there are no more unpleasant terms used than "dim" and "shabby;" likely symbolic of Florence's self-chosen future compared to the material wealth of her past.

Of the remaining novels, *Bleak House* has a brief description of the little church at Chesney Wold, and *Edwin Drood* (1870) depicts the interior and even the crypt of the cathedral at Cloisterham:

> An ancient city, Cloisterham . . . A monotonous, silent city, deriving an earthy flavor throughout from its Cathedral crypt, and so abounding in vestiges of monastic graves, that Cloisterham children grow small salads in the dust of abbots and abbesses, and make dirt-pies of nuns and friars (*ED*, 14).

There is, however, no pestilence or noxious effect noted from either the dust of the abbots and abbesses or from the "earthy flavour" of the place.

Burial Grounds

Far worse than the atmosphere in old churches was the ever-present danger to health engendered in the burying-grounds around them. The problem was addressed in the treatise mentioned above and about 1840 in an anonymous pamphlet published in London: "Horrors of London Burial Grounds being a Correct Account of the Horrible Disclosures made by Gravediggers, with the Manner of Cutting up Dead Bodies and other Horrible Transactions." Why such grisly occurrences were apparently commonplace was ascribed to the third motive cited by Bettesworth: dismembered bodies took less space, so more bodies could be interred in the same ground, generating more income for the sexton.

There were a number of mid-Victorian texts on intramural interment. George Alfred Walker, a surgeon, delivered a series of lectures on metropolitan graveyards. The lectures – of which Dickens had a copy[36] - were printed in full in the *Provincial Medical and Surgical Journal* (forerunner of the *British Medical Journal*) in 1840, Volumes 4 and 5. His *Gatherings from Grave-Yards, particularly those of London* appeared in 1839 and was carried in the *Westminster Review.*[37] Based on his research, a committee was appointed, W.A. MacKinnon as Chairman, leading to a report submitted in 1842 by Edwin Chadwick. The descriptions given by Walker and Chadwick are nearly identical to the burial ground where Nemo is buried in *Bleak House.*[38]

In 1842, there were 218 acres of intramural burial grounds in London alone, receiving some 40,000 bodies each year. The overcrowding was such that it was common in many burial grounds to burn coffins and destroy the bodies with lime. Still, Parliament did not act. MacKinnon, in *The Builder*, (3, 1845) gave notice that he would inform Parliament of the necessity of improving the health of towns by banning intramural interment. The reforms which he suggested were so extensive that it was claimed that better ventilation and draining of large towns were trifles by comparison.[39]

What finally turned the tide and set reforms in train was – once again – a cholera epidemic. Only then was the fact faced that the churchyards were overfull and simply no longer adequate. Further investigations were reported in *The Times* on October 8, 1849, which "brought to light more specific evils than those disclosed even by the researches which Mr Chadwick made by direction of the Government in 1842." A Bill was finally introduced on April 15, 1850 by Sir George Grey, the Home Secretary, to provide for interment in and near the metropolis. A Metropolitan Burial District was created by Act of Parliament, which granted the General Board of Health power to provide burial grounds and purchase the commercial cemeteries already in existence. *The Times* of May 4, 1850 commented on the Bill, lamenting the centralization which must be part of any such control, but that "[c]onsiderations of decency, economy, and health combine to enforce this reform upon us."

The 32nd clause of the Metropolitan Interments Bill, read in committee on June 11, 1850, dealt with the "Gain and Lucre" cited by Bettesworth, since it provided "compensation to the clergy for the loss of their present fees." Sir Benjamin Hall reported on burial practices at the church of St. Giles's-in-the-Fields, where

> It had been the practice . . . to make a feint of covering the coffin whilst the mourners were present; but as soon as they were gone, the body and coffin were taken up, the head of the deceased was severed from his body, and cast into a hole, in order

that putrefaction may speedily set in. This was done in order to afford more ground for burials, and to bring fees to the clergyman. [40]

This was certainly not to the liking of a certain group of men who make an appearance in one of Dickens's two historical novels, and to whom we now turn our attention.

Bodysnatching[41]

When we think of bodysnatchers in connection with Dickens, we of course think of *A Tale of Two Cities* (1859) and that "honest tradesman," Jerry Cruncher (Chapter 1, Book 2).[42] In line with the theme of the novel, Cruncher is a "resurrection man" – one of a league of men who disinterred newly-buried bodies to supply the anatomy theatres of hospitals and private anatomy schools with corpses for dissection. The need far outpaced the supply, since under a law of Henry VIII, only executed criminals could be dissected, intending less to further medical knowledge than to deny the wrong-doer a grave, which made dissection "a further Terror and peculiar Mark of Infamy."[43]

This is the law to which Dickens refers in *Nicholas Nickleby* when Squeers captures Smike in London:

> Where's the clothes you run off in? . . . Do you know that . . . it's a hanging matter – and I an't quite certain whether it an't an anatomy one besides (*NN*, 497).

In 1824, William Mackenzie published in Glasgow an "Appeal to the Public and to the Legislature on the necessity of affording Dead Bodies to the Schools of Anatomy by Legislative Enactment." Mackenzie pointed out that, under the current circumstances, "there is no other method of obtaining subjects but that of exhumation" and that the

> opposition which is made is made not against anatomy, but against the practice of exhumation: and this is a practice which ought to be opposed. It is in the highest degree revolting . . . [but] so long as no other means of procuring bodies for dissection are possible, it must be tolerated.[44]

While there were many even trivial crimes punishable by death, the sixteenth-century law limited the number of dissections to four a year, with the rights to the bodies assigned to the Company of Barbers and Surgeons – after 1742, to the surgeons alone. One suggestion for overcoming the deficit was to permit dissection of the unclaimed bodies of paupers who died in the workhouses. Henry Warburton, who headed a governmental inquiry into the running of schools of anatomy in 1829, put forward this suggestion, which was attacked by Thomas Wakley. He was against passing any law to regulate the dissection of the unclaimed bodies of the poor, . . . until so much of that statute which consigns the bodies of murderers to dissection shall have been repealed. . . . [N]o portion of the prejudice against dissection . . . will be removed, so long as it shall be deemed by the Legislature a fit punishment and degradation for the bodies of the worst of criminals.[45]

In *Our Mutual Friend,* Dickens makes oblique reference to this proposed source of corpses in the figure of Betty Higden, who is portrayed as one of the multitude who would rather die than go to the workhouse. She not only flees the workhouse as a dwelling, she sews sufficient money into the hem of her dress to pay for a proper burial. Whether, in fact, she does so out of fear of dissection, as stated by Lawrence Rothfield in his essay "Medical"[46] or simply out of fear of such a burial as described in both *Oliver Twist* (Chapter 5) and *Bleak House* (Chapter 11) is debatable. The one is no more horrible than the other.

The large number of bodies required for teaching purposes even led to the transportation of cadavers between England, Scotland and Ireland and finally moved Parliament to action. A Select Committee on the Teaching of Anatomy was convened in 1828. The work of this Committee resulted in the passage in 1832 of the Anatomy Act, which was designed by the utilitarian philosopher, Jeremy Bentham.[47]

Dickens refers directly or indirectly to the Anatomy Act in several places. First there is the scene at Dingley Dell, when Bob Sawyer and Ben Allen discuss "clubbing" for a subject (Chapter 30). In Chapter 31, Mr Pickwick asks Sam Weller if the man in the "celebrated sassage factory" was "burked" (*PP*, 379) - an expression which may be anachronistic. It refers to the murderers Burke and Hare – more accurately to their method of suffocating victims. They were active in Edinburgh between December 1827 and October 1828, and the term would not have been coined before their arrest. The narrated time has been identified as 1828, making the use questionable. M.J. Durey points out that "[i]ronically, Henry Warburton introduced his Anatomy Bill . . . into Parliament on the very day Burke was hanged in Edinburgh."[48]

Like the New Poor Law, The Anatomy Act, or "Dead Body Bill" as it was more commonly known, has been viewed as the "criminalization of poverty" and as "one of the most important indicators of the intensity of social tension in the Reform era."[49] Most of the public health issues of the age were related directly or indirectly to poverty – as indeed is often still the case in many areas of the world. There being little chance of escaping physically from poverty, brings us to the attempt to escape at least temporarily by chemical means.

Substance Abuse

Medically speaking, substance abuse refers to use or extent of use other than intended of any chemical substance, such as alcohol or narcotics. The subject is not usually one mentioned in connection with Dickens and public health, but from today's perspective, it clearly belongs in that constellation.

Alcohol

One widely-discussed and hotly-debated issue in the nineteenth century was the use and abuse of alcohol. One of the causative factors can be seen in the Beerhouse Act of 1830 under which beer duty was abolished and sales permitted to any ratepayer for two guineas excise and certain securities. The result was 44,134 *new* beerhouses within the following six years.[50] In competition to these came the Gin Palaces or "Gin-Shops," as Dickens called them in a sketch published in the *Evening Chronicle*, which expressed "outrage at what he considered misguided attitudes to drink."[51] An interesting comment from the text connects these places with poverty:

> Although places of this description are to be met with in every second street, they are invariably numerous and splendid in precise proportion to the dirt and poverty of the surrounding neighbourhood. The gin shops in and near Drury Lane, Holborn, St. Giles's, Covent Garden, and Clare Market, are the handsomest in London. There is more of filth and squalid misery near those great thoroughfares than in any part of this mighty city (*SB,* 182).

Even as early as 1835, Dickens was championing the poor and speaking out against the Temperance Societies:

> Gin drinking is a great vice in England, but wretchedness and dirt are a greater; and until you improve the homes of the poor, or persuade a half-famished wretch not to seek relief in the temporary oblivion of his own misery, with the pittance which, divided among his family, would furnish a morsel of bread for each, gin shops will increase in number and splendour. If Temperance Societies would suggest an antidote against hunger, filth, and foul air, or could establish dispensaries for the gratuitous distribution of bottles of Lethe water, gin palaces would be numbered among the things that were (*SB*, 185).

The Temperance Movement, which culminated in the Prohibition of the 1920s in the United States, was based on the theory that "alcohol itself has an habituation potential; everyone can become aggressive and behave badly. In short, anyone who consumes alcohol risks his personal integrity and delivers himself up to the demon alcohol."[52] Apart from journalistic pieces like the one cited above, Dickens satirized the movement – and its association with evangelical fundamentalism - in a number of novels; Mr Stiggins of the *Pickwick Papers* comes immediately to mind as an early example.

Dickens's portrayals of drinking range from the innocuous to the catastrophic in an approximate parallel to the overall "darkening" development in his novels discussed in Chapter 1. While the *Sketches* do include Gin Shops, drinking and even drunkenness in *Pickwick Papers* – though frequent – is mostly harmless, with the abusive form of alcohol consumption limited to interpolated stories like the dying clown.

Alcohol, mostly as social drinking, appears in all of Dickens's novels. Some characters abuse alcohol: Dick Swiveller (*OCS*), whose alcohol consumption may have predisposed him to the pneumonia which nearly killed him; Agnes Wickfield's father (*DC*) becomes alcoholic largely due to the machinations of Uriah Heep, but is saved by Micawber and, of course, by Agnes, his "angel in the house." Important characters who abuse alcohol and do not recover are Mr Cleaver (*OMF*), who is a study of delerium tremens and death due to alcohol abuse[53] and the stonemason Durdles (*ED*), whose drunkenness gives Jasper opportunity to obtain the key to the cathedral crypt.

This frequent literary use of alcohol was a source of distress to the "tee-totalers" who abstained from all use of alcohol, including Dickens's former illustrator, George Cruikshank.[54] Dickens defended his portrayals in several letters, one of which will serve as representative of his opinion. On September 1, 1842, he wrote to a New York merchant, Jacob Harvey, that

> It is commonly one of the weaknesses of my characters that they drink spirituous liquors – just because that is one of the weaknesses of real men. . . . I certainly do not advocate Temperance Doctrines, and on this plain ground; my reason and sense of justice are not at all convinced that men who can drink without abuse and excess should be deprived of the enjoyment of drinking in moderation because there are a vast number of men in the world who do not know what moderation is. A great many good qualities and a great many genial feelings are brought out in good men by a cheerful glass. I think Temperance may be as immoderate and irrational in its way as abuse is in ITS way; and what is called Total Abstinence is, in my opinion, a good thing ridden to death – just as Drunkenness is.

The Lancet obviously agreed, stating that "the assertion made by teetotalers that alcohol is poisonous in all doses is rank quackery."[55]

What may be less known than the Temperance Movement is the concurrent increase in the use of "medicinal" alcohol. According to *The Lancet* of February 11, 1865

There are few things more remarkable in the recent history of medicine than the extent to which alcohol has been introduced, and the importance which has been attached to it in the treatment of disease. Coincidently with a greatly reduced use of it in society has occurred a greatly increased use of it in medicine. Judging from the London practice of the last few years, a cursory and casual observer might think that alcohol was a remedy of specific power, the triumphant introduction of which was to make Dr Todd as famous as vaccination made Jenner, or chloroform Simpson.

That Dickens was aware of this development can be seen in Chapter 48 of *Bleak House*. Allan Woodcourt has returned to London and meets Jenny and Jo. The latter is obviously very ill and Woodcourt takes it upon himself to buy him some bread– which he can't eat, being "so sick and miserable, that even hunger has abandoned him." Then

Allan looks about for an apothecary's shop. There is none at hand, but a tavern does as well or better. He obtains a little measure of wine, and gives the lad a portion of it very carefully. He begins to revive, almost as soon as it passes his lips. (*BH,* 584)

It is this medicinal use of alcohol, even for children and adolescents, which perhaps surprises modern readers most. But apparently Dickens was simply describing common medical practice.

Opium

In 1851, a letter signed "Medicus" appeared in *The Lancet,*[56] which leads into another problem with substance abuse, namely that of opium. The writer points out that

Since the crusade of the teetotalers against spirit-drinking, there is a great reason to believe that the practice of taking opium is on the increase; and when one of the first of our physicians describes it as a virtuous and comparatively harmless species of excitement compared with gin drinking, I cannot but think he treats it with undue levity and may unintentionally contribute to the extension of the vice.

Opium played a greater role in Victorian life than we might suppose. It was available in a variety of forms:

opium pills ..., opium lozenges, ..., opiate confection, . . . opium liniment . . . There was the famous tincture of opium (opium dissolved in alcohol), known as laudanum, which had widespread popular sale, . . . The dried capsules of the poppy were used, as were poppy fomentation, syrup of white poppies and extract of poppy. There were nationally famous and long-established preparations like Dover's Powder, that mixture of ipecacuanha and powdered opium originally prescribed for gout by Dr Thomas Dover, the medical man and student of Thomas Sydenham. . . . The children's opiates like Godfrey's Cordial . . . were long-established. They were everywhere to be bought. Until 1868, there were no bars on [the retailing of opium] at all (and even after 1868 restrictions were still quite minimal).[57]

Even in medical circles the addictive properties were not clearly understood. The drug was prescribed for a wide variety of illnesses, including dysentery, asthma, diabetes, malaria, cholera and as general pain relief (see Chapter 2, "Renal colic"). A manuscript review in *The Lancet* points out that the "treatment of fever by opium is not . . . to supersede other remedies which may be specially required to combat concurrent symptoms – wine, brandy, diffusible stimulants when exhaustion takes place . . . " and that opium "in suitable doses [is not] in anywise contraindicated for children suffering from fever."[58]

It is interesting that this widespread use of opium in Britain was not the cause of the Opium War with China in 1840-42.[59] Still, Jeremy Tambling writes that in *Dombey & Son*

> Walter Gay and Florence go to China immediately after they are married. The context of this is the British-Chinese Opium War of 1840 . . . Florence's honeymoon on a ship to China would have been spent amongst quantities of opium.[60]

This is likely incorrect, since ships carrying opium to China did not sail from England, but only from India. Nor would the opium have been brought by ship from China, since most of the opium entering Britain was actually from the Middle East and came overland. The fleet involved in the opium trade consisted of special ships which plied solely between India and China, operated by the East India Company, which had the monopoly.

Although opium is involved with the plot of *Edwin Drood*, smoking, as depicted there, was less common in England than the various "cordials" and therefore less relevant to the public health question. *Bleak House* comes to mind in connection with opium, as one of many of the issues at least mentioned in the novel. Esther's father, Captain Hawdon, dies of an overdose of opium – whether intentional or not is left unanswered. What surprises is that Hawdon's supplier was Allan Woodcourt (Chapter 11). This appears to have been nothing out of the ordinary, since "a little opium more or less, is nothing" to the "unmoved policeman" on his rounds. Nonetheless, John DaCosta writes in 1905 that "it grates upon us to reflect that [Woodcourt] sells opium to habitués".[61]

Dickens's use of opium smoking and the opium den in *Drood* is traced to visits he made to such a place "at around the time he was writing the first chapter and, in all probability, at earlier dates also."[62] Once *Drood* brought opium dens into a broad popular consciousness, they became part of the literary repertoire, for example in novels by Wilkie Collins and later Oscar Wilde. *Edwin Drood* is the "first example of a subgenre of the double-life tale in which a specific association is made between opium dens and Oriental ambience and the protagonist's shift between identities."[63] Indeed, there is a passage in DeQuincey's *Confessions of an English Opium Eater* which would appear to have coloured much of the theme in *Drood:*

> Southern Asia, in general, is the seat of awful images and associations. As the cradle of the human race, it would alone have a dim and reverential feeling connected with it. But there are other reasons. No man can pretend that the wild, barbarous, and capricious superstitions of Africa, or of savage tribes elsewhere, affect him in the way that he is affected by the ancient, monumental, cruel, and elaborate religions of Indostan &.[64]

As the mechanisms behind the effect of opiates became known and the dangers of addiction were recognized, more stringent laws were passed. The use of opium disappeared from the pages of "romance" to take its place in the pages of twentieth-century crime novels, reflecting the fact that only medically-controlled applications are now permissible under the law.

Conclusion

The Lancet of November 4, 1865 carried an article entitled "Our Mutual Friend" which is appropriately excerpted here, since it supports the view that Charles Dickens was not only popular as a writer, but also powerful as a force in social reform.

> We look back upon these reports as among the most useful of the public services which it has been our privilege to render. We are especially glad to find at our side Charles Dickens, the earnest and warm-hearted opponent of social tyranny, one of the truest and most powerful friends of the oppressed, whether in middle or lower ranks of life.

While many of the issues addressed by Dickens and the *Lancet* are no longer relevant in England to the same degree, they remain so in much of the world today. Diseases, particularly those of poverty like cholera, considered eradicated in Western countries, are still prevalent in developing countries and others, like tuberculosis, are once again ravaging the populations where sanitation remains – or has again become – a problem. Read in this light, Dickens's novels are just as relevant now as they were more than a century ago.

Turning from public to general family health, we will now have a look at the remedies common in Dickens's day. Some of these are still known, most of them have been replaced by more sophisticated – usually chemical – means, while others are even making something of comeback.

[1] Cited in Briggs (1985) 260.
[2] Berridge in Webster (1995), 70.
[3] Much of Dickens's concern is voiced in his journals; see Appendix 4 for pertinent articles.
[4] Rosenberg (1983), 40.
[5] Michael Slater, Introduction to the Penguin Edition (1971), 138.
[6] Slater (1971), Note 13, 263.
[7] Dombey Sr. reminds one of Henry VIII in his obsession to have a son to carry on the "dynasty". This is underlined by Mrs Skewton's references to Henry VIII.
[8] Fildes (1986), 58.
[9] *Gummi - Die elastische Faszination* - Ausstellung des Deutschen Hygiene-Museums, Dresden. Berlin (1995), 310. My translation.
[10] Letter dated January 26, 1837; published in *The Dickensian*, May 1967, 68:77.
[11] Footnote 1 to Chapter 2, Penguin Edition cites this as "Queen Charlotte's Lying-In-Hospital in Marylebone Road, an institution which also sent out foster-mothers to nurse children." The hospital is now Queen Charlotte's and Chelsea Hospital.
[12] Rose (1986), 50.
[13] Fildes (1986), 169 and 175.
[14] Grant (2000), 21. Dickens would undoubtedly have agreed; the redheads in his works are undesirable characters –like Fagin (*OT)* or Uriah Heep (*DC)*.
[15] Rose (1986), 21.
[16] Fildes (1986), 53/4.
[17] Ste. Marthe, Paedotrophiae, cited in Fildes (1986), 188.
[18] Ibid, 100.
[19] Ibid, 55. This device was used as late as World War II in Germany.
[20] Charles Dickens and W.H. Wills. "Received a Blank Child". *HW* (1853), 7: Interesting to note is the institution of a "baby box" in Hamburg, Germany in January 2000, since the number of abandoned babies has increased despite readily-available contraception and legal abortions.
[21] A popular "stress management" course in Germany recently advised counting – Mr Meagles's advice to Tattycoram is apparently appropriate after all!
[22] Dorothy Porter, in Bynum and Porter (1993), 1241.
[23] Norris Pope, "public health, sanitation and housing" in Schlicke (1999), 471.
[24] Fielding (1988), 106.
[25] *Ibid*, 129. Compare this with "There is not a drop of Tom's corrupted blood but propagates infection and contagion somewhere."(*BH*, 575), written at about the same time.
[26] Pope, in Schlicke (1999), 469.
[27] 1778-1861, Lord Mayor 1832. See Fielding (1988), 108.
[28] Fielding (1965) I, 113.
[29] Oppenlander (1984).
[30] *AYR*, 7:303.
[31] *HW*, 8:526.
[32] Bettesworth (1721), 40.
[33] Ibid,56.
[34] Ibid, 59.
[35] That he was concerned with the problem is evidenced in two *Uncommercial Traveller* essays published in *AYR* III, p. 85 "City of London Churches" and *AYR* IX, p. 493, "The City of the Absent".
[36] *Letters*, 6, fn 47.
[37] 1842, No. 37, 210-16.

[38] See Chapter 11, 139; Chapter 16, 207. Activities of the "Mrs Jellybys" of the day were also commented by Walker in his 4th lecture in denouncing philanthropy which looks for objects of sympathy on the banks of the Niger and ignores poverty at home. See also Slater, *Journalism*, 108: Dickens's review in the *Examiner* of a Niger expedition.
[39] Curl (1972), 197.
[40] *Household Narrative*, June 1850, 127.
[41] There is extensive literature available on bodysnatching; see for example Howell (1926).
[42] Lyn Pykett (2002) sees Cruncher as part of Dickens's contrast between Paris, the "city of spectacle, a public theatre on whose stage the drama of history is enacted before a participatory mass audience" and London, a "quiet, polite and private city, whose citizens – from the gentlemanly Mr Lorry to the comic-grotesque Resurrection Man, Jerry Cruncher – pursue their avocations conscientiously and in an orderly manner" (Pykett [2002], 163).
[43] Richardson (1987), 37.
[44] Mackenzie (1824), 30.
[45] *The Lancet*. June 5, 1829.
[46] Rothfield, (1999), 77.
[47] Marshall (1999), 17-21.
[48] Durey (1976), 204.
[49] Richardson (1987), 192.
[50] Carter, E. (1933).
[51] Schlicke, "Sketches by Boz" in Schlicke (1999), 531.
[52] Vogt (1981), 217. My translation.
[53] The German medical historian von Engelhardt apparently has trouble with the translation: he reports an "alcoholic child" in *OMF*, not realizing the parent/child inversion involved. von Engelhardt (2000), 147.
[54] See "Fraud on the Fairies," *Household Words*, (1953) 8:97.
[55] Dr Glover on "The Philosophy of Medicine". *The Lancet*, February 15, 1851.
[56] *The Lancet* (1851) I:694.
[57] Berridge (1999), Part II, section 3.
[58] William Tutin Haycraft. *On the Use of Full doses of Opium in Fever*. Reviewed in *The Lancet* (1851) I,:363.
[59] There is extensive literature available on the subject; see for example: Fay (1975).
[60] Tambling (1993), 311.
[61] DaCosta (1905), 12.
[62] Schlicke (1999). *The Mystery of Edwin Drood:* sources and content, 393.
[63] Milligan (1995), 110.
[64] DeQuincey (1867), 87.

CHAPTER 8: Folk Medicine, Unorthodox Medicine and Superstitions

In Chapter 2, various diseases which Dickens uses were reviewed in relation to the respective novel and their medical reception. We now turn to remedies which he cites. Writing in 1983, the historian Charles Rosenberg describes the then growing interest in past medical care. One consequence of this interest, he says, is

> the awkward realization that the larger part of such care provided to the sick has always been offered by individuals who did not consider themselves and were not considered by their contemporaries to be physicians.[1]

There were a number of books on home doctoring in Dickens's time, and Rosenberg states that

> No single health guide before the twentieth century enjoyed a greater popularity than William Buchan's *Domestic Medicine*. Between the 1769 publication of its first edition in Edinburgh and the appearance of its last English-language version just over a century later in Philadelphia, Buchan's *Domestic Medicine* appeared in at least 142 separate editions. [2]

That Dickens knew this book – or at least knew of it – is reflected in Chapter 16 of *Little Dorrit:*

> When [the Meagles family] went away, [the housekeeper, Mrs Ticket] always put on the silk-gown and the jet-black row of curls … established herself in the breakfast-room, put her spectacles between two particular leaves of Doctor Buchan's *Domestic Medicine* and sat looking over the blind all day until they came back again. It was supposed that no persuasion could be invented which would induce Mrs Tickit to abandon her post at the blind, … or to dispense with the attendance of Dr Buchan; the lucubrations of which learned practitioner, Mr Meagles implicitly believed she had never yet consulted to the extent of one word in her life (*LD,* 192).

Since Dickens was a novelist of broad appeal, who incorporated many popular ideas and beliefs into his works, folk remedies might be expected to play a role, and this is indeed the case. Beyond bleeding the patient,[3] little is told of what the medical men did when they were called in. But cases of illness or injury for which no medical man was consulted are to be found, and with them, remedies applied by laymen.

As in the review of diseases, this chapter makes no pretensions of being complete. I have selected the examples on the basis of their apparent familiarity among nineteenth-century laymen, as implied from Dickens's texts. Most of these remedies have been discarded, but some are still known, though perhaps little used, and still others are reappearing in current practice.

Folk Medicine

Treatment of Bruises/Black Eyes

The first layman offering a remedy is Jingle in *Pickwick Papers*. Mr Pickwick writes notes on the cabman's report of the great age of the horse, his diet and so on. In a scene which appears to have inspired the opening scene of Bernard Shaw's *Pygmalion*, a row ensues, which is terminated by Jingle. Taking Pickwick and his friends into the travellers' waiting room, Jingle calls to the waiter:

> 'Here, Waiter! . . . raw beef-steak for the gentleman's eye, - nothing like raw beef-steak for a bruise, sir; cold lamp-post very good, but lamp-post inconvenient – damned odd standing in the open street half-an-hour, with an eye against a lamp-post – eh' (*PP,* 9).

Here Dickens cites two bruise remedies: raw beef and cold, the latter of which he typically exaggerates to the ludicrous by choosing a common but hardly practicable "applicator" and presenting the suggestion in Jingle's identifying, disjointed speech.

The beefsteak remedy is applied also in *David Copperfield.* David fights the butcher's boy – and loses the first time. Agnes, the angel in the Wickfield house, is instinctively a good nurse, and puts ". . . beef-steaks . . . to [David's] eyes" and rubs the bruises "with vinegar and brandy" (*DC*, 219). Using beef as a remedy for injuries inflicted by a butcher's boy sounds a bit on the homeopathic principle of "like cures like" and possibly Dickens was writing tongue-in-cheek here, though the remedy was common and is still known.

Vinegar

Used as reported by Agnes, vinegar was apparently a frequently-applied bruise remedy. This is because, on evaporating from the skin, vinegar "steals" the warmth from the area to which it is applied, making it a crude form of cryotherapy. It is very often reported by Dickens in conjunction with brown paper. One scene in which this remedy features largely is found in Chapter 34 of *Nicholas Nickleby*. Mr Squeers tells Ralph Nickleby that, after the attack by Nicholas, he was like "a large brown paper parcel, chock full of nothing but groans" (*NN*, 61).

Another proponent of vinegar and brown paper is Fascination Fledgeby in *Our Mutual Friend.* Fledgeby wants information from Jenny Wren concerning Lizzie Hexam's whereabouts. She arrives at Fledgeby's just as Alfred Lammle is leaving. Lammle had thrashed Fledgeby, and Fledgeby asks Jenny to apply vinegar and brown paper plasters to the bruises on his back. Jenny does so – but with a twist: she adds pepper. This could be attributed to Jenny's usual show of aggression – and could be related to Foetal Alcohol Syndrome, if Dr John Cosnett's recent retrospective diagnosis is correct.[4] But Fledgeby has alienated Jenny from her friend, Riah, and has uncertain designs on Lizzie. Jenny has mistrusted him – rightly[5] – and Dickens let this act of aggression be more a justified act of retaliation and retribution, not only for Jenny herself, but also for the others wronged by Fledgeby.

The miasma theory of epidemic diseases justified the widespread use of vinegar, to which an anti-miasmic property was attributed. Due to the belief that disease originated from vapours arising from the soil, and particularly from damp marshes, anything which made any attempt to mask the airborne odour would be credited with a degree of curative or preventive powers, much as amulets were thought to ward off other evils. By carrying nosegays and strewing herbs or vinegar, one had the illusion of taking some precautions – and inhaling the fragrance of flowers was in any case preferable to the stench of sickrooms, jails, ships, hospitals or other crowded places.

In *The Old Curiosity Shop*, one of the first things Dick Swiveller notices on regaining consciousness after about three weeks is that "the atmosphere was filled with a cool smell of herbs and vinegar" (*OCS*, 491). In *Bleak House*, Harold Skimpole recommends sprinkling a little vinegar in the room where the sick crossing-sweeper, Jo, is put for the night. In *A Tale of Two Cities,* this same precaution is taken in the court where Charles Darnay is tried for espionage: "The court was all bestrewn with herbs and sprinkled with vinegar, as a precaution against gaol air and gaol fever" (*TTC*, 94).

No vinegar is mentioned in the court scene in Chapter 56 of *Great Expectations*, but it is mentioned in passing that the sheriffs carry nosegays and the court is strewn with herbs: "The sheriffs with their great chains and nosegays. . ." (*GE*, 339).

Edgar Rosenberg, editor of the Norton edition, points out that

> The nosegays and flowers the Judge and other high-court officials carry on them, as well as the herbs strewn about the court … are vivid reminders of the noxious stench emanating from the Newgate prison cells next door and the constant threat of contagion – a virulent form of typhus – to the Old Bailey. The prophylactic was

generally adopted after an epidemic of jail fever in 1750 had killed the Lord Mayor of London, his aldermen, the jury, and spectators.[6]

Vinegar also makes its appearance as a restorative, especially for fainting women. So, for example, even the dim-witted Edmund Sparkler of *Little Dorrit*, knows the value of aromatic vinegar, because his mother used it.

It is seen that laymen made common use of an everyday substance, one readily found in every household, especially in days when preserves were made at home. Vinegar is coming back into current use today in certain fashionable diets, and its value as an environmentally-sound cleanser is also gaining in recognition.

Sal Volatile/Hartshorn/Smelling Salts

Another very popular restorative, especially for sensitive females, was sal volatile, more commonly known as smelling salts. Dickens knew the less common term, as Sam Weller of *Pickwick Papers* illustrates. Ben Allen thinks Bob Sawyer should marry his sister, Arabella, who, however, marries Nathaniel Winkle. Mr Pickwick goes to break the news to Ben and Bob, and finds Ben's aunt already on the scene, since she was informed by Arabella herself in a letter. On hearing the news, Ben Allen becomes violent, which alarms the old lady, causing her to faint. She is forgotten on the arrival of Mr Pickwick and Sam Weller until Sam says:

> Here's a wenerable old lady a lyin' on the carpet waiting for dissection, galwinism, or some other rewivin' and scientific inwention (*PP*, 604).

He then tells the boy employed by Sawyer to "bring out the wallatilly!" Janet Oppenheim points out that "Dickens, always in touch with the state of popular information about science and medicine, knew that electrotherapy ("galvanism" after the Italian physicist-physician Luigi Galvani (1737-1798)) was familiar enough to the reading public to enjoy a little fun at its expense."[7]

Nicholas Nickleby has a number of fainting women and the terms sal volatile, hartshorn and smelling salts are all used. Miss Knag, termed a "fright" and an "elderly person" by some of Madame Mantalini's customers who prefer to be assisted by the young and beautiful Kate Nickleby, terminates her patronizing "protection" of Kate and has hysterics. When Kate returns to the work area, she finds Miss Knag being treated with "hartshorn, vinegar, and other restoratives, . . . having fainted desperately" (*NN*, 226).

In Chapter 14, Nicholas and Smike arrive at Newman Noggs's to ask his help. A neighbour, Mr Crowl, intruding on an anniversary party at the Kenwigs's, says he hopes the two have not come from any jail or hospital and brought a fever. The thought causes Mrs Kenwigs to faint and Mr Kenwigs

> held a fat smelling-salt bottle to his lady's nose, until it became a matter of some doubt whether the tears which coursed down her face, were the result of feelings or *sal volatile* (*NN*, 180).

Mrs Kenwigs appears to have been particularly susceptible to overreaction. Her Uncle Lillyvick later marries Miss Petowker and apparently disinherits the Kenwigs's children. Miss Petowker deserts her husband and elopes with a half-pay captain, and the crushed Mr Lillyvick returns home. On his appearance in the Kenwigs's home,

> the emotions of Mrs Kenwigs became so violent, that Mr Kenwigs was fain to administer hartshorn internally, and vinegar externally, and to destroy a staylace, four petticoat strings, and several small buttons (*NN*, 689).

Another histrionically-talented woman is Mrs Varden, the locksmith's wife in *Barnaby Rudge*. As frequently the case among Dickensian women, her hysterics are self-willed and a means of controlling her family. Varden suggests an outing, whereupon his wife bursts into tears, resulting in

> much damping of foreheads, and vinegaring of temples, and hartshorning of noses and administration of stimulants of which Miss Miggs herself partook as a preventive measure (for fainting is infectious) (*BR*, 205).

The administration of diverse remedies and the language in which Dickens describes the procedure offers an interesting commentary on the behaviour of at least certain types of women. The remedies are apparently to be administered only by a sympathetic woman; certainly not by the husband, whose submission was the object of the exercise. It is known, of course, that fainting was considerably more common then than now[8] and that it played a role in the "war of the sexes," including the struggle for dominance in the family.

Josiah Bounderby in *Hard Times* finds himself in the potentially awkward position of telling his housekeeper, Mrs Sparsit, that he is going to marry Louisa Gradgrind and arms himself with

> a bottle of the strongest smelling-salts. 'By George,' said Mr Bounderby, 'if she takes it in the fainting way, I'll have the skin off her nose, at all events!' (*HT*, 138-9)

This is typical Bounderby; he knows that Mrs Sparsit doesn't like Louisa and possibly hoped to become Mrs Bounderby herself, but his will is all that matters.

One especially hypochondriacal female is Herbert Pocket's Aunt Camilla in *Great Expectations*. She is one of Miss Havisham's toadying cousins and reports at length on the malaise she undergoes by being so "affectionate and sensitive," and "what ginger and sal volatile [she is] obliged to take in the night" (*GE*, 71). Later, when Joe tells Pip that Miss Havisham has died of the injuries suffered in the fire, Pip asks about her property. It would appear that Miss Havisham had a sense of humour after all. She left Camilla the perfect legacy: "five pound fur to buy rushlights to put her in spirits when she wake up in the night," as Joe reports (*GE*, 346). They may, however, be unnecessary, since the expection of an inheritance from Miss Havisham was the apparent basis of her "affection"/affliction.

A typical Dickensian description of common human behaviour in an emergency is given in Chapter 46 of *The Old Curiosity Shop*. Nell and her grandfather have unexpectedly met the poor schoolmaster again. Nell faints and is carried to a small nearby inn, where everyone present mills around, expecting someone else to do something. Only the landlady acts, and brings "a little hot brandy and water, . . . vinegar, hartshorn, smelling-salts, and such other restoratives" (*OCS*, 355). Here, the use of restoratives does not serve to emphasise what Dickens sees as ridiculous or manipulative female behaviour. Nell is exhausted and in the early stages of tuberculosis.[9] Dickens has created a pathetic heroine, who is intended to elicit pity and concern. The landlady is therefore not catering to whims, but behaving as expected of a "good nurse = good woman". It is possible to postulate that the "merits of the case" were – at least in part – financial in nature. But it remains that the landlady does act, which no-one else does.

Cold water

Cold water alone is also found as a remedy for fainting. Sometimes the application is gentle, as in the case of Florence Dombey and Captain Cuttle. Florence, struck by her father, flees the house, turning to the only friend she knows, Walter Gay's uncle, Sol Gills, at the Wooden Midshipman. Florence runs into the shop and promptly faints.

> Captain Cuttle snatched from his breakfast table a basin of cold water, and sprinkled some upon her face (*DS*, 707).

The more common application is less considerate. When Oliver Twist is "restored" to Fagin, Nancy becomes enraged and faints, and her friend, Miss Betsy, "opportunely arrived to throw water over her friend ..." (*OT*, 105). In *The Old Curiosity Shop,* one can easily imagine the import of Quilp's hint to his mother-in-law, Mrs Jiniwin, that "there was abundance of cold water in the next apartment" should she feel faint (*OCS*, 45). Throwing cold water over an unconscious person remained part of the folk canon for some time, its popularity undoubtedly aided by its appearance in older films, but it was actually not only folk medicine, as attested to in an article in the *Lancet* of April 13, 1839. William F. Barlow, Esq. reported on "A Case of Epilepsy," saying: "I dashed cold water in the face, knowing this to be beneficial in convulsive affections of an epileptic kind but I did not find it of advantage here."

Cold remedies

The first mention that someone will catch cold calls for prevention rather than remedy. The Pickwickians are invited to spend Christmas at Dingley Dell with the Wardle family. Among the amusements is a skating party, which terminates abruptly when Mr Pickwick breaks through the ice. He is wrapped in three or four shawls, runs back to the house, gets into bed while Sam lights the fire in his bedroom. Punch was made after dinner – three bowls – and Pickwick escaped taking cold

> which proves, as Mr Bob Sawyer very justly observed, that there is nothing like hot punch in such cases: and that if ever hot punch did fail to act as a preventive, it was merely because the patient fell into the vulgar error of not taking enough of it (*PP*, 373).

The cold remedy *par excellence* is reported in *Nicholas Nickleby*. Pyke and Pluck appear on the morning after Mrs Nickleby has accidentally met Sir Mulberry and Lord Frederick Verisopht at Ralph Nickleby's, ostensibly to inquire whether she had taken cold going home. In a typical Mrs Nickleby monologue, she describes the following cure:

> You have a gallon of water as hot as you can possibly bear it, with a pound of salt and six-pen'orth of the finest bran, and sit with your head in it for twenty minutes every night just before going to bed; at least, I don't mean your head – your feet (*NN*, 345).

Mrs Nickleby's mode of speaking makes this remedy appear absurd, since it obviously had nothing whatever to do with her getting over a cold lasting from Christmas to April. But Mrs Nickleby was not the only Dickensian character to use this or a similar remedy. In *Hard Times,* Mr Bounderby's recommendation to Mrs Sparsit is to "put [her] feet into the hottest water [she] can bear, and take a glass of scalding rum and butter after [she gets] into bed" (*HT*, 260). Dickens himself applied this remedy as well. In a letter to Catherine in October 1835 he asked if it remained damp and foggy, whether Catherine would "advise [him] to stay at home, take some gruel, try hot water for [his] feet, and go to bed early?"[10]

Bounderby's suggestion of rum was also apparently a Dickens household remedy. On December 27, 1846, Dickens wrote to Forster that he was going to "take a jorum of hot rum and egg in bed immediately and to cover [himself] up with all the blankets in the house."[11]

None of the cold remedies known to Dickens worked for him during his second trip to the United States in 1868. He took cold soon after arrival and it persisted until he left the country again. He wrote to Forster on January 5 that he had "tried allopathy, homœopathy, cold things, warm things, sweet things, bitter things, stimulants, narcotics, all with the same result. Nothing will touch it."[12]

Even today, of course, there is no "cure" for a cold. Modern remedies may alleviate the symptoms, but the folk saying still applies: a cold will last 7 days with medication or a week without it.

Sherry and egg

Cousin Feenix in *Dombey and Son* recommends "the yolk of an egg, beat up with sugar and nutmeg, in a glass of sherry, and taken in the morning with a slice of dry toast." (*DS*, 912) if Dombey is feeling weak after the collapse of the House. Feenix appears here to be describing a pre-Victorian "cure" for a hangover, which was not Dombey's problem, of course. But that was not the only use for the remedy. In *Little Dorrit,* Bishop says that as a young man, he had often felt overtaxed and the "yolk of a new-laid egg, beaten . . . with a glass of sound sherry, nutmeg and powdered sugar, acted like a charm" (*LD*, 247).

This was apparently another household remedy in the Dickens family. In a letter to Georgina from New York about his reading tour in January 1868, Dickens reports being debilitated by fatigue and the persistent cold mentioned above and that he had "established the custom of taking an egg beaten up in sherry before going in, and another between the parts." [13]

Brimstone and treacle / Tar-water

Two last "remedies" remain to be mentioned. Each appears in only one novel without reference anywhere else in Dickens's writings. Remembering the days when cod-liver oil was popular as a "tonic" and preventive for practically everything, it is quite plausible that these concoctions were used for self-medication more than one might think.

Brimstone and treacle

The Master and Mistress of Dotheboys Hall were, on their own testimony and advertisement, solicitous of the health of the boys entrusted to their care. One measure for promoting health was the administration, at regular intervals, of brimstone and treacle (or in the US, sulphur and molasses). Mr Squeers, still trying to make a reasonable impression on Nicholas on his first day at Dotheboys Hall, says it's to "purify their blood." Mrs Squeers is more honest:

> Oh! Nonsense! . . . They have the brimstone and treacle, partly because if they hadn't something or other in the way of medicine, they'd always be ailing and giving a world of trouble, and partly because it spoils their appetites and comes cheaper than breakfast and dinner. So, it does them good and us good at the same time, and that's fair enough, I'm sure (*NN*, 86).

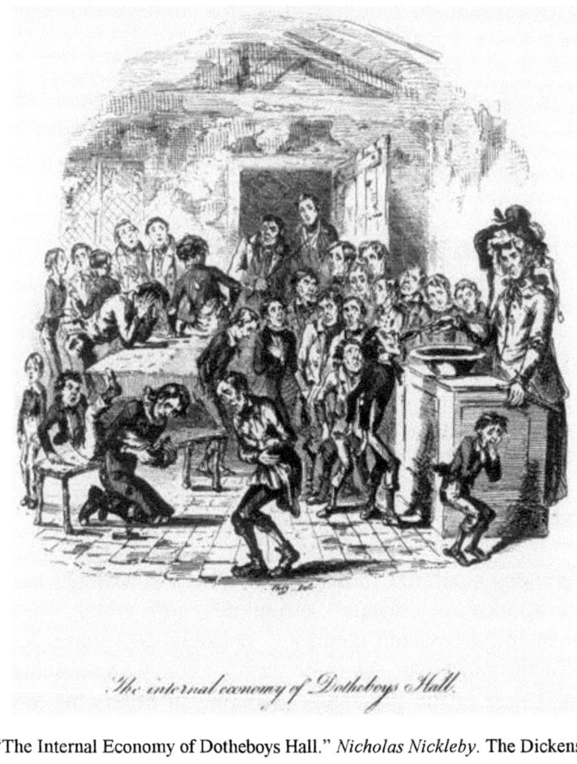

Fig. 9: "The Internal Economy of Dotheboys Hall." *Nicholas Nickleby.* The Dickens Museum.

In a clear act of just retribution, the boys "dose" Mrs Squeers herself when it becomes known that Squeers has been jailed.

An explanation for this mixture can be found, for example, in a Victorian domestic encyclopaedia called *Enquire Within upon Everything*. This book was published in many editions – the 62nd in about 1880 by Houlston & Sons, London. It lists sulphur and flour of brimstone as laxatives. Another popular household book, Mrs Beeton's, published initially in 1861, cited sulphur and treacle as a cure of ringworm. Knowing the miserable diet given the boys at Dotheboys Hall, occasional doses of this mixture may even have been justified.

Tar water

In *Great Expectations*, Mrs Joe's remedy for nearly any malady or misdemeanour (other than the "Tickler") appears to have been tar-water "having a belief in its virtues correspondent to its nastiness" (*GE*, 16).

Edgar Rosenberg explains in a footnote that this combination of pine extract and fir extract, was

> the most widely touted panacea of the eighteenth century, thanks to Bishop Berkeley (1685-1753), who, in his essay *Sirus: A Chain of Philosophical Inquiries Concerning the Virtues of Tar Water* (1744) claimed it as a cure for nearly everything.[14]

Realizing just how nasty tar water was makes the *Schadenfreude* even greater when Uncle Pumblechook swallows some which Pip had unwittingly put into the brandy bottle.

As different as these two "remedies" are, the grounds for their administration in the novels are similar: the exercise of power over weaker individuals was a considerably stronger motive than any benefit which resulted – or even could have resulted – from the "medicine."

Unorthodox Medicine

There are references scattered throughout Dickens's writings to what are now considered unorthodox or "fringe" disciplines and which were not entirely orthodox even in the nineteenth century.[15] Dickens uses these descriptively and humourously for the most part. In some cases, Dickens commented in letters on his belief or disbelief of the principles involved, in others his attitude might be inferred from the use he makes of the practice.

In a chapter entitled "Early Victorian Radicals and the Medical Fringe," the historian J.F.C. Harrison states that a "preliminary check shows at least ninety individuals . . . having associations with both social reform and fringe medical movements."[16] It is thus not unlikely that some of Dickens's friends and acquaintances, especially Dr John Elliotson (1791-1868), introduced him to these movements.

Homœopathy

One of the approaches considered unorthodox by Dickens's contemporaries was homœopathy, discussed in connection with the "Mudfog" sketches in *Sketches by Boz.*[17] While others of the Victorian "fringe disciplines" have all but been forgotten, homœopathy is currently enjoying a revival due to its holistic approach and its basis in natural plant medicines as opposed to man-made pharmaceuticals. Although acquainted with Frederick Hervey Foster Quin, who founded the London Homœopathic Hospital, Dickens apparently didn't take homœopathy seriously. His main use of homœopathy is as a definition of anything very small, such as in the example of the workhouse diet cited from the *Sketches* and in the "homœopathic doses" of food and drink which Noah Claypole gives Charlotte in *Oliver Twist* (*OT*, 287).

Mesmerism

The discipline in which Dickens most firmly believed is mesmerism. Introduced in 1775 by the German physician Franz Anton Mesmer (1734-1815) in Vienna, this was originally a "magnetic cure" using steel magnets,

> by which elevation of the general well-being, eradication of pain and abnormal movements, and suppression of sensory perceptions could be achieved; it progressed to the point that [Mesmer] could exercise a healing influence on the sick person by means of his will.[18]

The scientific mesmerists believed that receptive individuals could be mesmerized through special techniques of concentration. This could be beneficial in surgery, since there was no anaesthesia, and in various nervous illnesses. Dr Elliotson's unorthodox ideas, particularly his support of mesmerism, resulted in his resignation from the University Hospital in London in 1839. His reputation with respect to mesmerism was such that Thackeray could say in *Vanity Fair (1847)* "As Alexis, after a few passes from Dr. Elliotson, despises pain . . ."[19] and know that his readers would understand the allusion. Dr Elliotson wrote Dickens in May 1841 inviting him to a demonstration of mesmerism to be held at Elliotson's house.[20] What appealed especially to Dickens was that "[m]esmeric operators, putting their subjects into trance, had the opportunity to be physicians of the mind, special benefactors of mankind."[21]

In an article in 1851 on "Philosophy of Medicine," Dr Robert M. Glover comments on the "extreme amount of caution which is required before we give our consent to such marvels."[22] Dickens's opinion differs, as is clearly expressed in his own activities and also in a letter to Henry Morley dated January 9, 1836, in which he expressed his belief in mesmerism and his disbelief in homœpathy. His interest and activities have been thoroughly documented in several biographies.[23] The appearance of mesmerism in Dickens's fiction is the issue in question at the moment.

In his book *Dickens and Mesmerism,* Fred Kaplan discusses Dickens's use of mesmerism and mesmeric vocabulary. Considering mesmerism to be a means of discovering self, Kaplan sometimes, however, quotes out of context. For example, he writes "One can in moments of insight discover one's self; there is such a self to be discovered by 'a magnetic and instinctive consciousness'"[24] and attributes the quote, correctly, to *Martin Chuzzlewit*, Chapter 8. The quotation originally, however, reads: "The parlour was wainscoted, and communicated to strangers a magnetic and instinctive consciousness of rats and mice" (*MC* 126). Kaplan has thus taken a quotation concerning realisation by association of things *outside* one's self and applied it to cognizance of self, which is questionable. Actually – a most rare occurrence – I would here question Dickens's choice of words. While "animal magnetism" may be a facetious reference to mice, I would question a consciousness of mice as being "instinctive," since the association between the sound behind the wainscoting and the mice is learned.

Emphasising Dickens's interest and the general interest in mesmerism in the Victorian Age, Kaplan tends, in my view, to overdo his interpretations. Every time any character exerts ascendancy over any other, Kaplan claims the ascendant character has mesmeric powers. He postulates mesmerism as a source of Quilp's mastery over his wife, and in the relationships between Gashford/Lord George Gordon and, in turn Gordon/crowds, Mr Carker/Rob the Grinder,[25] Mr Tulkinghorn/Lady Dedlock; he relates it to visions both direct and reflected and generally gives it credit/blame for actions and reactions. The most obvious use of mesmerism is John Jasper's approach to Rosa Bud, and I would agree that this is indeed the case. Rosa, speaking to Helena Landless says that Jasper has "forced her" to understand him, and that she is frightened (*ED*, 53). The description given is certainly of consciousness against one's will, which could be postulated as the correlate of unconsciousness against one's will.

The other instances postulated by Kaplan are power struggles, which can be interpreted as such without recourse to magnetism. Quilp's mastery over his wife is attributed to sexual prowess – and undoubtedly fear of his sadistic pleasures. Gashford manipulates Gordon by repeating the family motto, but this is an appeal to pride and perceived duty rather than a trance-inducing mantra; Gordon fires the crowd by addressing a topic made volatile by recent legislation and prejudice. Mr Carker terrifies Rob, so even if his teeth are the bright objects which might mesmerize, they simply emphasise his predatory and dangerous nature. Tulkinghorn feels his power when he lets Lady Dedlock know that her story has been discovered and if she reacts as if in shock (trance-like state), this is small wonder. Mesmeric influences are not necessary in these characters. Dickens might also have been reluctant to describe the use of mesmeric influences mainly for evil purposes, knowing that these fears were rampant in society at the time, and applying his own mesmeric powers for good. While Kaplan sees mesmerism with evil, selfish, or manipulatory intent as ubiquitous, beneficial mesmerism appears to be lacking in his view. He sees Dickens as a "novelist who could use the mesmerist's emphasis on will, energy and mind as intensified metaphors for his exploration of the condition of man."[26] Whether will, energy and mind were stressed *only* by mesmerists in the early Industrial Revolution is questionable, since these attributes form no small part of the Protestant work ethic, and Dickens, even had he known nothing of mesmerism, was a man of strong will, enormous energy and powers of mind.

My opinion is supported in an interesting two-part article published in *The Dickensian.* Arthur Cox, editor of the Penguin Classics Edition of *Drood,* contests Kaplan's use of "will" and "will power" in connection with mesmerism, citing Kaplan's statement that 'To the mesmerists, the faculty that controls this universal fluid is "will" or "will power."' In Cox's view, this statement

> would be impeccable if he dropped the last three words. . . . Mr Kaplan's preoccupation with 'will power' leads him sadly astray when he considers Dickens's novels. He takes every mention or display of will, or power, or resolve, assertion, domination, and so on, as betraying the presence in the story of mesmerism, and, not surprisingly, he finds a good many instances.[27]

Whether Cox himself overdoes the interpretation of mesmerism in *Drood* is an open question. Not only will he have Jasper mesmerizing Rosa, but Neville Landless, who helps murder Edwin and then takes the blame, and Canon Crisparkle, who goes for an inexplicable reason to the Weir and finds Edwin's watch. At any rate, we quite definitely have an instance of mesmerism by Jasper, and if Cox's theory is correct, a consciously malevolent use. Cox is convinced that the reason why the role of mesmerism has only been discussed in connection with *Drood* is that it is the *only* novel by Dickens in which mesmerism has any role to play.

Mesmerism went out of fashion, partly due to the attacks launched by Wakley in the *Lancet.* For example, there was an advertisement in the Table of Contents for the *Lancet* of January 4, 1845:

> In consequence of some Recent Publications, THE LANCET will contain a COMPLETE CRITICAL HISTORY, commencing in January, of THE RISE,

PROGRESS, AND MOCK MARVELS OF THAT HALLUCINATING FRAUD, known by the term "MESMERISM."[28]

Perhaps contributing more to its demise was the discovery and introduction of anaesthetics. As Winter says, "[r]ather than being exposed as fraudulent or explained away by progressive science, it was absorbed into other practices, particularly psychic research, physiology and psychoanalysis."[29] It remained part of theatrical presentations during the early to mid-twentieth century, then practically disappeared. It is noted, however, that mesmerism is once again under discussion for use in place of anaesthesia, particularly in dentistry, and that it has re-entered the world of (extremely dubious) entertainment as a feature of a television show. On a more serious level a demonstration was held recently at the Open University's Department of Psychology. Also, Robin Waterfield recently published *Hidden Depths: the Story of Hypnotism*. In a review in *The Lancet*, Sue Kinder of the School of History, Classics and Archaeology, Birkbeck College in London concludes by saying that "Hypnosis has a colourful history and Waterfield tells a remarkable tale, but he is unlikely to make many converts."[30] Nonetheless, a sports column by Christopher Clarey in the *International Herald Tribune* of March 26, 2003 reports that the American figure skater Michael Weiss is undergoing "hypnotherapy". The therapist Topher Morrison, speaking of the stereotypes associated with hypnotism, is quoted as saying:

> It's from the stage shows; the spooky stuff. People think they are going to be made to quack like ducks and bark like dogs. But that is slowly stepping aside, and people are starting to realize it's a powerful tool.

Recent research performed in Montreal, Canada, has also reportedly brought evidence that hypnosis has a real effect on the physiological response to pain.[31] So whether we will see a resurgence of hypnotism in medicine remains to be seen.

Phrenology

Proposed as a "bold attempt to detach the understanding of the mental functions from philosophy and root it in anatomy," phrenology was supposedly the physiology of the brain, which was considered as divided into areas, each area controlling a particular character trait or physiological system. The size of such an area, as palpable on the skull, directly indicated "the power or lack of it for the faculty in question."[32] At about the time Dickens began writing, phrenology was beginning to enjoy considerable popularity, which lasted until the advent of neurology and physiology in the second half of the nineteenth century. Its popularity did not always guarantee favourable reception and opinions varied widely as to whether phrenology was to be considered a science, a pseudoscience or pure humbug. The phenomenon originated in Vienna, and *The Lancet* published a series of five articles beginning June 25, 1836 under the heading: "Lectures on Phrenology" by F.X. Broussais (1772-1838), a leading figure at the University of Paris medical school. We can use an excerpt of a report from *The Lancet* as an example of a phrenological report:

The Examination of Fieschi's Head

The forehead is moderately developed, and the facial angle is also moderate. The cranium is very long, and the temples are remarkably flattened. They do not present any trace externally of the organs of *murder*, "*ruse*", or *ponderance*, but the organ of *theft* is very well marked on the superior median line. The organs of *benevolence* and *theosophy* are evident. The organ of *firmness* is not well-marked, and that of *vanity* and *pride* still less so. The same remark applies to the organs of *courage* and *attachment.*[33]

This article was a detailed account of the principal circumstances connected with an autopsy. Fieschi was not identified in the article,[34] but one sentence toward the end of the article may give a clue: "… it appears as if its cellular tissue was penetrated with numerous air-bubbles, in the same way as the pia mater in all criminals who are executed." From the "findings" of the autopsy, a phrenologist might surmise that Fieschi was a man executed for theft, but that turns out to be not quite correct: Fieschi was a Corsican executed for an assassination attempt on King Louis Phillipe of France in July 1835. He died protesting that he was "a great criminal, not an assassin!"[35]

One proponent of phrenology was Dickens's close friend, Dr Elliotson, who spoke at the first meeting of the Phrenological Society of London. Referring extensively to the writings of Gall,[36] he raised the question of "how any one, who has studied Gall, and examined for himself into the facts of the coincidence of development and character, can doubt the truth of phrenology."[37] Another interesting statement in defence of phrenology is made by E.J. Hytch in *The Lancet* of 1837-38, who writes that Phrenology is essentially a science of observation. "To observation alone are we indebted for the establishment of a science … which is destined to effect a moral revolution in society."[38] Attempts were made to include phrenology in the curriculum of medical education, but it

remained too controversial and never succeeded in establishing itself as a reputable science. It was, in its way, a clumsy step in the direction of the modern recognition that different faculties are controlled by separate areas of the brain.[39]

If Hytch were correct in saying that phrenology is "a science of observation," one might expect Dickens, a most observant man, to be an adherent. Also, considering that phrenological adherents were "at the forefront of mid-century agitation for social and legislative change, using its doctrines as a platform from which to fight for reform in penal institutions and lunatic asylums…"[40], we might expect to find Dickens among the number. But, unlike Goethe, who "took phrenology so seriously . . . that he once would not allow a satire on it to be performed at Weimar,"[41] George Eliot, who "shaved her head to undergo phrenological reading,"[42] or Charlotte Brontë, whose "letters and fiction [use] the vocabulary of phrenology to dramatize the possibilities of psychological transcendence of social limitations",[43] Dickens seems not to have taken phrenology seriously. His use of phrenology in the novels is openly facetious, for example in *Martin Chuzzlewit*, in which Pecksniff's fall led to to the "development of an entirely new organ, unknown to phrenologists, on the back of his head" (*MC*, 10). In *Little Dorrit*, Dickens clearly allies phrenology with humbug. Christopher Casby, father of Arthur Clennam's old love, Flora, is considered by all to be a benevolent man, with his reputation based on his appearance: "So grey, so slow, so quiet, so impassionate, so very bumpy in the head ..." (*LD*, 139) Casby is, of course, anything but benevolent. He lets his front man, Pancks, take the blame for brutality in collecting rents in Bleeding Hearts Yard – until Pancks revolts, tells the truth about the "Patriarch" and subjects Casby to the indignity of having his hair cut off in front of the tenants, reducing his benevolent appearance to its bare truth as well.

In Dickens's treatment of phrenology, the humour is satirical. As Tytler points out,

> Dickens implies that the cult of phrenology is quite as stupid as are many other Victorian cults he attacks in his novels. This is amply suggested in *Edwin Drood*, where a satirical thrust at phrenology occurs, appropriately enough, in the context of a dig at one of the author's pet aversions: philanthropy.[44]

We know now that phrenology did not cause the great social revolution predicted by Hytch. This was expected by its detractors, such as Dr Robert M. Glover, in the article cited in connection with mesmerism, who accused the phrenologists of taking "note of all positive facts" and disregarding the rest. According to the *Bibliographisches Lexikon*, it was especially the lay interest and misappropriation of Gall's teachings that kept phrenology from being taken seriously, since

> it was abused directly as a sort of oracular art and promulgated for mercenary motives even by those who didn't believe in the truth of it. But it would be a grave injustice to count Gall himself among this sort of charlatan and swindler.[45]

Superstitions

Superstitions in medicine do not appear to play much of a role in Dickens's works. One might have expected to find such things in the early works, associating less sophistication and maturity with such matters. This turns out to be an erroneous assumption. The superstitions which are found are in *David Copperfield, Bleak House,* and *Our Mutual Friend.* Their scarcity is also somewhat surprising when we realize that Dickens had a copy of *On Superstitions connected with the History and Practice of Medicine and Surgery* by Thomas Joseph Pettigrew in his library at Devonshire Terrace in 1844 – the year the book was published. Since Dickens was not involved in editing at the time, it could not have been a review copy which he had been sent in connection with any journal or newspaper, so the fact that the book was in his possession would seem to indicate Dickens's personal interest. In *All the Year Round,* [46] there is an article entitled "Medical Nuts to Crack" which concludes with a tale from Pettigrew's book.

The superstitions which Dickens used were fairly well-known in the nineteenth century. From Dickens's use, it would appear that he did not, himself, grant them much credence – if any – but wove them into his descriptions for humorous purposes.

Caul

David Copperfield begins with several superstitions. David reports that the nurse and "some sage women in the neighbourhood" declared that he would be unlucky and would see ghosts, since he was born on a Friday night. David further reports that he was born with a caul, which "was advertised for sale, in the newspapers, at the low price of fifteen guineas." (*DC*, 1) According to E. and M.A. Radford, [47] *The Times* of May 8, 1848 advertised a caul for sale at six guineas, so fifteen was apparently a high, rather than low price. A caul is part of the foetal membrane which sometimes adheres to the infant's head at birth. Old wives' tales assert that a child born with a caul cannot drown. Trevor Blount, editor of the Penguin Edition, footnotes "caul" and says that this is "an obvious hint in *David Copperfield* that the hero will eventually find happiness and not share Steerforth's fate."[48] Blount may be correct in the latter part of his interpretation, though there is never any danger of David's drowning, while the first part contradicts the "sage women" in the village.

Death and the tide

There is another superstition connected with mariners in *David Copperfield.* Barkis is ill beyond medical help: Mr Chillip says that "the College of Physicians, the College of Surgeons, and the Apothecaries' Hall…couldn't help him. He was past both Colleges…and the Hall could only poison him" (*DC*, 359). The only question is when the man will die. Peggotty's brother tells David that Barkis is "going out with the tide" and explains that "people can't die along the coast except at low tide, nor be born except at high tide." Barkis revives enough to recognize David, says – as he had done as a marriage proposal to Peggotty – 'Barkis is willin', then, the reader is told, "it being low water, he went out with the tide" (*DC*, 364).

Drowning

Our Mutual Friend, in which the river plays such a major role, also contains references to superstitions around drowning. Rogue Riderhood, who is an exceptionally unpopular character on the waterfront, having stolen from a living sailor (dead ones didn't count, since only living men can be said to own anything or have any use for possessions), is run down in his boat by a steamer. He is brought in to the Six Jolly Fellowship Porters, where one of the regular customers tells the doctor that the body should be hung up by the heels, then rolled over a cask. The doctor, however, prefers artificial respiration. Later, Riderhood attempts to blackmail Bradley Headstone, knowing that Headstone not only attempted to murder Eugene Wrayburn – which he would willingly have ignored and even applauded – but attempted to throw suspicion on Riderhood – which was another matter. Headstone attacks him at the lock and Riderhood says it won't do any good, since "a man as has come through drowning can never be drowned." But Headstone can be, and manages to hold Riderhood and disprove the superstition.

Cramp bone

Sairey Gamp's imaginary friend, Mrs Harris, in *Martin Chuzzlewit* carries an odd collection of things in her pocket. When Sairey asks that tea be made, and buttered toast be served she says that Mrs Harris carries with her some teeth, which Mr Gamp had knocked out, along with "two cramp-bones, a bit o' ginger, and a grater like a blessed infant's shoe, in tin, with a little heel to put the nut-meg in ..." (*MC*, 705) Cramp-bones were sheep's kneecaps, which were thought to prevent cramps. Ginger was often used for treatment of indigestion (see Herbert Pocket's aunt, Chapter 8 above); nutmeg is mentioned above in connection with egg beaten in sherry and may have been kept handy for that reason.

Other cramp-bones are found where one might expect them; in small boys' pockets. Prince Turveydrop's apprentices kept "string, and marbles, and cramp-bones in their pockets" (*BH*, 495). It might be assumed that the cramp-bones were kept to avoid cramps in overexerted calf-muscles if the boys had to dance a great deal. By putting them in ignorant boys' pockets, however, Dickens points to the ridiculousness of the superstition.

Conclusion

The above review demonstrates, in parallel to the various illnesses which Dickens observed and described, his knowledge of the remedies and applications common to his day. Some of these remedies have gone out of style – at least in Western cultures medicine is more sophisticated than ever and patients more educated as well. A major factor is undoubtedly also the emergence of health insurance or national health services, which guarantee access to adequate health care for at least a large segment of the population. It is, perhaps, well to remember that medicine had not finished its development to a modern science[49] and that the profession was divided both in training and inclination at the time Dickens was writing. Still, Dickens's lay knowledge accurately reflects practices of his day and, as has been demonstrated, some of these practices were his own. He mentions the superstitions cited in this section only to ridicule them.

There is one issue which is now considered a superstition, but which was viewed differently well into the nineteenth century. This is spontaneous human combustion, which plays a prominent role in *Bleak House*. Literary criticism has dealt with its metaphoric role, largely to the exclusion of the forensic side of the question. As the following will show, the chapter is not even yet closed.

---

[1] C. Rosenberg (1983), 22.
[2] Ibid, 22.
[3] Bleeding a patient and applying leeches are making something of a comeback in very specific situations; see: *The Lancet* (1998), 352.S4, 2014: "Why leeches influence my physical examination" by Shetal Shah. There was also a program on German television on the efficacy of bleeding (Aderlaβ) in prevention of stroke. ["Die Visite" on 6.2.2001, North German regional television (N3)].
[4] See Chapter 5.
[5] Dickens describes Fledgeby as having very small, close-set eyes – as mentioned in connection with blindness, always a bad sign for a Dickens character.
[6] *Great Expectations*, Norton edition (1999), footnote 3, 339.
[7] Oppenheim (1991), 119. Sam also speaks of "dissection" – the second reference to this topic in *PP*, cf. Chapter 7 above.
[8] The question of tight stays as a factor may be raised but ignored, since in scenes like the one quoted here, Dickens's women characters "faint" voluntarily.
[9] See Chapter 5.
[10] *Letters*, 1, 85.
[11] *Letters*, 4, 686.
[12] Forster (1899), II:411.
[13] Quoted in Forster (1899), II:415.
[14] Norton edition (1999), footnote 6, 16.
[15] See Bynum and Porter (1987) for a discussion of orthodoxy in medicine.
[16] In: Bynum and Porter (1987), 198.
[17] See Chapter 1.

[18] *Bibliographisches Lexikon hervorragender Ärzte aller Zeiten und Völker*, 4, (1908), 179-81 (my translation).
[19] Thackeray (1983 reprint), 269. Interesting to note, this is where the term "make a pass at someone" comes from.
[20] See *Letters*,2:148.
[21] Kaplan (1988), 183.
[22] *Lancet*, 7, February 15, 1851, 36.
[23] For example Forster (1899): I, 189 and II, 70; Ackroyd (1990): 243-5, 366, 448-51 573.
[24] Kaplan (1975), 233.
[25] L.D. Browning's article on mesmerism in Schlicke (1999) 375 also postulates "a form of mesmeric power" for Quilp and Carker.
[26] Kaplan (1975) 234.
[27] Cox, A.J. (2000), Part 1, 150, footnote 63.
[28] Written by Charles Radclyffe Hall, MD, extra-licentiate of the college of Physicians, London, the series actually started on February 1, 1845. The capitalization is in the original text.
[29] Winter (1998), 8.
[30] Kinder (2003), 1992.
[31] Smith, Michael (2003), 21.
[32] Loudon (1997), 239.
[33] *Lancet* (1835-36), II:75, original italics.
[34] It would not have been necessary at the time.
[35] See *AYR,* 17:322, 30. March 1867.
[36] Franz Joseph Gall, (1758-1828) German-born French physician and founder of phrenology.
[37] Quoted in *The Lancet* 1837-8, I:295-298, here 295.
[38] *Lancet,* 1837-38, II:29-30.
[39] Gilmour (1993), 139.
[40] Shuttleworth (1996) 63.
[41] Tytler (1982), 96.
[42] Winter (1998), 9.
[43] Shuttleworth (1996), 66.
[44] Tytler (1982), 263.
[45] *Bibliographisches Lexikon der hervorragenden Ärzte aller Zeiten und Völker*. (1908) 671, my translation.
[46] July 6, 1861, 5:358-60. Author unidentified.
[47] *Encyclopaedia of Superstitions.* 1961, 92-3.
[48] Note 1 to Chapter 1, 951.
[49] See Bynum (1994) for general information.

CHAPTER 9: Spontaneous Human Combustion

As discussed in the preceding chapter, one might expect a medical layman to use undefined malaise and superstitions more than recognizable diseases and even more that medical curiosities would play a large role in Dickens's works. His interest in the unusual, the abnormal, the grotesque has been the subject of innumerable articles and books. There are, however, relatively few such medical curiosities appearing beyond brief mention in the novels. The one topic which is used as a major component, and which is still subject to controversy and difficult to categorize, is spontaneous human combustion (SHC). A chapter is devoted to this topic because Dickens's use of SHC caused considerable controversy – both during his lifetime and since – and because of its rather unique status as an entity or non-entity. What makes it even more compelling is the fact that fairly recent books and articles have been written *supporting* the existence of the phenomenon. Both traditional reports and recent books are presented, but the discussion still ends with a question mark.

The best-known reference to SHC in Dickens's works is in *Bleak House*, but there are a few earlier instances. For example, Chapter 11 of *Martin Chuzzlewit* tells of a serenade at Mrs Todger's boarding house, which was so dismal that "If the two Miss Pecksniffs and Mrs Todger had perished by spontaneous combustion," it couldn't have been worse (*MC*, 187). Published in the same period, *A Christmas Carol* also mentions SHC: Scrooge, waiting for the appearance of the second Spirit was "apprehensive that he might be at that very moment an interesting case of spontaneous combustion, without having the consolation of knowing it" (*Carol*, 86). As Trevor Blount points out, these instances are witty. "Yet, implicit all the time is the assumption that spontaneous combustion is perfectly possible."[1]

Again, the most famous is the following passage from *Bleak House* when Weevle goes downstairs to meet Krook at the appointed time, finds him not there and recruits Guppy as reinforcement.

> The cat has retreated close to [the door], and stands snarling - not at them; at something on the ground, before the fire. . . .
>
> Here is a small burnt patch of flooring; … and here is - is it the cinder of a small charred and broken log of wood sprinkled with white ashes, or is it coal? ..... O Horror, he **is** here! and this from which we run away, is all that represents him.
>
> Help, help, help! come into this house for Heaven's sake!
>
> Plenty will come in, but none can help. The Lord Chancellor of that Court, true to his title in his last act, has died the death of all Lord Chancellors in all Courts, and of all authorities in all places under all names soever, where false pretences are made, and where injustice is done. Call the death by any name … it is the same death eternally - inborn, inbred, engendered in the corrupted humours of the vicious body itself, and

that only - Spontaneous Combustion, and none other of all the deaths that can be died (*BH*, 416-418).

This description of Krook's death is, as Dickens himself indicates in the final paragraph, a particularly apt metaphor. Chancery and its minions, attacked strongly throughout the novel as an institution devoted to the devouring of wealth and - much worse - of the health and sanity of those who become entangled in its web, must at some point self-destruct. The "corrupted humours" which power the functions will eventually result in the destruction of the vessel. Krook, the "Lord Chancellor" of the collected detritus of defunct existences, is the aptly-named symbol.

Non-human spontaneous combustion

But what of the phenomenon itself? Spontaneous combustion of hay and silage, oily rags and paper resulting from the heat generated by rapid oxidation of their components has been well-known for centuries. For example, the "fire from heaven" reported in the Old Testament (I Kings 18) is interpreted by Michael Harrison[2] as spontaneous combustion.

In Exodus 3:2, we find the account of the angel appearing to Moses in a bush which "burned with fire [but] the bush was not consumed." The similarity with lack of damage to the surroundings in the historical reports of SHC is striking and such references would likely have occurred to Dickens's Bible-literate contemporary readers.

Dickens made one reference to non-human combustion in his *Sketches by Boz:* "The Streets – Morning", in which the servant wishes "that the principle of spontaneous combustion would extend itself to coals and the kitchen range" (*SB*, 52). One might ask why Dickens's didn't use spontaneous combustion *per se* instead of the more controversial spontaneous *human* combustion. After all, Chancery was the institution, not the Chancellor; and the shop was a likely place for spontaneous combustion. The answer is, perhaps, that Dickens believed in SHC, that it *is* controversial and infinitely more horrifying than common spontaneous combustion and also, had the rag and bottle shop burst into flame, Miss Flite and the surrounding neighbourhood would have been endangered.

What modern readers tend not to realize in reading *Bleak House* (unless they read Dickens's Preface to the book version of August 1853) is the fact that spontaneous combustion of the *human body* occupied a considerable space in scientific literature of the eighteenth and nineteenth centuries. An "impressive mass of historical precedence" had been reported by Claude-Nicholas le Cât (or Lecat)[3] in Rheims in 1725. But the earliest full account of the phenomenon which I have found appears to have been that in *De Incendiis Corporis Humani Spontaneis*, published in Leyden by Jonas Dupont in 1763.

Dickens's use of the phenomenon was attacked immediately after publication of the part, leading him to the defense made in the Preface to the 1853 book version. The controversy between George Henry Lewes and Dickens has been extensively documented and need not be reiterated here.[4]

In the preface of 1853, Dickens writes that "there are about thirty cases on record" (*BH*, vi). This agrees reasonably well with the twenty-eight cited as having been "documented between 1468 and 1806"[5] of which 16 were reported in France and 22 with the prolonged use of alcohol.

Dickens cites the various cases of which he had read and ends by stating that he champions "no hypothetical explanation of the fact."[6] He does not mention that he consulted his friend, Dr John Elliotson and borrowed from him the manuscript of a lecture Elliotson had given on the subject. The manuscript which Dickens borrowed has apparently not survived, so we cannot know what Elliotson wrote. It is, however, evident from Dickens's letter dated February 7, 1853 that Elliotson believed in the phenomenon and provided what Dickens considered conclusive arguments:

> It is inconceivable to me how people can reject such evidence supported by so much familiar knowledge and such reasonable analogy. But I suppose the long and short of it is, that they don't know, and don't want to know, any thing about the matter.[7]

Historical records

We don't know what Elliotson wrote, or even exactly what "sources" Dickens consulted, but we do know some of the historical reports to which Dickens refers. One case which is cited in nearly all accounts of the phenomenon is that of Mary Clues or Clewes, a widow of Coventry, who was said to have drunk up to a quart of rum each day. She was found totally consumed except for her legs and one thigh (*Annual Register*, 1775). Another case involved an Ipswich fisherman's wife who - as reported by Dickens in his letter to Lewes - had "drunk an immense quantity of spirits within a few hours of her death."

One of the more widely-publicized accounts is that concerning the Countess Cornelia Bandi, written by the Rev. Joseph Bianchini, a Prebend in the City of Verona, translated and published in the *Philosophical Transactions* of 1745. All that remained of the Countess was her head, two legs untouched to the knee and three fingers. It should be noted that the Countess, unlike the other two women, was not an habitual drunkard. But immoderate use of alcohol was always cited as one of the common factors. For example, the "Literary Gazette" for June 28, 1828 discusses spontaneous human combustion and reports that

> a memoire lately read to the Académie des Sciences completely establishes the fact and states the . . . principle circumstances attending it, derived from chemical and medical observations on no fewer than fifteen cases of its occurrence.

The first of these "principle circumstances" was immoderate use of alcohol.

Michael Harrison, writing 151 years after the article in the "Literary Gazette" identifies the following factors which are almost invariably included in the historical reports:

(1) the victim is a chronic alcoholic
(2) a lamp or other source of ignition is always present
(3) the victim is usually an elderly woman
(4) the victim is solitary or at least dies alone.

Harrison also identifies findings at the scene which distinguish SHC from natural fire:

(1) there is little damage to surroundings
(2) there is a residue of greasy ashes
(3) the body is almost totally consumed
(4) the extremities often escape serious burning.[8]

In Krook's case, the only things at odds are his gender and that his extremities did not escape. He was almost always drunk and mention is made of the "bottle so rarely absent from the table"; "there is a very little fire left in the grate"; Krook was socially isolated and distrustful of people; there is "a small burnt patch of flooring"; and all that remained of him was "a small charred and broken log of wood sprinkled with white ashes, or is it coal?"

Obviously Dickens knew the factors in the reports and took pains to include them both in his description of the socially isolated, habitually drunken Krook while alive and in his description of Krook's death.

Dickens's defense is now *generally* accepted as absurd. Certainly literary critics have adopted this opinion. But as I will discuss below, there are other people who believe not only in the *possibility*, but indeed in the *veracity* of the event.

Medical writings on SHC and Medical Jurisprudence

The *British Medical Journal* of March 19, 1870 discusses an article in the *British and Foreign Medico-Chirurgical Review* by a Dr Alexander Ogston on the "truth of spontaneous combustion of the human body." Dr Ogston reports that his researches

> prove that there can be no doubt that weight of authority is in favour of spontaneous ignition, or, at least, of increased combustibility - two modes of viewing the subject, which have been generally combined under the title of spontaneous combustion, or *empresmus.*[9]

He goes on to discuss the theories (including gas accumulation with ignition by electricity within the body, and alcohol) and concludes by stating that

> the recorded cases which can be looked upon as reliable countenance no such doctrine as spontaneous combustion, but point merely to increased combustibility on accidental ignition.[10]

But that does not mark the end of the medical discussion. *Anomalies and Curiosities of Medicine*, published in 1896, contains about three pages of text on SHC in a chapter headed "Physiologic and Functional Anomalies". The text begins:

> Spontaneous combustion of the human body, although doubted by the medical men of this day, has for many years been the subject of much discussion; only a few years ago, among the writers on this subject, there were as many credulous as there were skeptics. There is, however, no reliable evidence to support the belief in the spontaneous combustion of the human body. A few apocryphal cases only have been recorded. [11]

The text goes on to repeat some of the cases, notably that reported by Bianchini on Countess Bandi, and the murder case of the Countess von Görlitz, in which the German chemist, Baron Justus von Liebig (1803-1873), was consulted. In investigating the case, Baron von Liebig and the anatomist Dr Theodor Ludwig Bischoff (1807-1882) performed the first experimental attempts to reproduce the phenomenon under controlled conditions. The experiments failed to show that flesh steeped in alcohol will burn. According to Harrison "Liebig accepted the fact of death by spontaneous combustion, but firmly rejected the theory (current even today) that indulgence in alcohol was a predisposing factor."[12]

With no less a figure than Justus von Liebig involved in the investigation of a murder which was to be passed off as spontaneous human combustion, it seems reasonable to expect some mention of the phenomenon in texts on medical jurisprudence. Two nineteenth-century texts on medical jurisprudence published in England bear this out. The first is *Medical Jurisprudence* by JA Paris, MD, FRS, FLS and JM Fonblanque, published in 1823. These authors consider the term "spontaneous human combustion" to be incorrect, for in every recorded instance, the approach of some burning body, as that of the flame of a candle, or an ignited pipe, appears to be necessary for its occurrence.[13]

It is noted that the phenomenon *per se* was not rejected. Indeed, the authors quote Dr Gordon Smith[14] as saying that

It can no longer be doubted, that persons have retired to their chambers in the usual manner, and in place of the individual, a few cinders, and perhaps part of his bones, were found.[15]

Several sources of case reports are cited, including twenty-eight cases in Plouquet's *Literatura Medica*, a "considerable number" in Dr Trotter's "Essay on Drunkenness", and a French *Dictionnaire des Sciences Médicales*. An explanation, attributed to two French doctors Dr Fodéré and Dr Marc [16] is that this species of spontaneous combustion is "due to the united action of hydrogen and electricity in the first instance, favored by the accumulation of animal oil and the impregnation of spirituous liquors."[17]

The circumstances surrounding the incident are the same as those cited from Harrison above, with the exception of the claim that the body does *not* ignite spontaneously. The conclusion drawn is that

If the bodies were actually found consumed, in the manner described, it is quite impossible to suppose that they were burnt by ordinary means. . . . [A]t a period when criminals were condemned to expiate their crimes in the flames, it is well known what a large quantity of combustible materials was required for the burning.[18]

A degree of skepticism is, of course, apparent: "*If* the bodies were actually found consumed. . ." The text does not give any information on how to prove or disprove the matter.

Charles Meymott Tidy, MB, FCS published a second text in London nearly forty years later, in 1862. In *Legal Medicine* Part I, Chapter XI is headed "Combustibles and Explosives" and pages 533-535 are devoted to "Spontaneous Combustion of the Human Body". The article begins:

There is no subject in the whole range of Medical Jurisprudence on which so much romance has been built as this. Since 1692, when the subject was first seriously discussed, popular novelists have often embellished their works by the introduction of some spontaneous combustion story, or amused themselves by telling or re-telling some of the current legends on the subject. The disappearance of the law-writer *[sic]* in Dickens's *Bleak House* is perhaps one of the best of these.

Briefly mentioning writers on medical jurisprudence, the author draws the conclusion that "there are no authentic cases of true 'spontaneous' combustion of the human body on record." Since, however, there are numerous cases on record in which persons have met their death by fire under unusual circumstances, Tidy further concludes that "the body of drunkards, especially if corpulent, is more than ordinarily inflammable" and that a slight accident could possibly cause ignition. Like the earlier work, Tidy refers to Dr Marc, among others, and presents the same summary of conditions. One interesting comment which he makes - indicative of the progress of scientific investigation, no doubt - is that

> Most of the recorded cases, it must be admitted, are marred by a want of precision, or by an evident credulity on the part of those who relate them. And not a few of the supposed cases of spontaneous combustion turn out to be murders, in which the culprits hoped to conceal the traces of their crime by fire.

Two recent twentieth-century books on forensic pathology mention SHC. The older of the two, *Forensic Pathology* by Dominick J. DiMaio, a retired Chief Medical Examiner in New York City, and Vincent J.M. DiMaio, Chief Medical Examiner and Director Regional Crime Laboratory in San Antonio, Texas, include spontaneous human combustion in a section on death in flash-fires. The section concludes:

> This section would not be complete without mention of spontaneous human combustion. This phenomenon and/or concept is absurd and warrants no further discussion.[19]

A British counterpart, also entitled *Forensic Pathology*, describes some "very strange instances of fatal burning" and the author admits to having seen "a pair of undamaged house slippers, with feet still within, the legs burned off at ankle level and no remaining body above…" The article continues:

> It seems extraordinary that virtually a whole adult body can be consumed, including the skeleton, with minimal surrounding fire damage, but many such cases are on record and have helped to substantiate the myth of 'spontaneous human combustion.'[20]

The author, Dr Bernard Knight, a Professor of Forensic Pathology, attributes these cases to the "wick theory," in which body fat burns slowly, using the clothing as a wick, like a candle flame. This is one of many theories, and is the one espoused by Michelle Phillips, a freelance writer for the *Medical Post Canada* in an article "History of the Human Candle" published on January 28, 2003. One theory relates "the practice of ingesting gunpowder in tea and tonics in the eighteenth and nineteenth centuries" as contributing to combustion and explaining the "timeline of the phenomenon."[21] There are two illustrations accompanying the article: one is, of course, from *Bleak House*.

Literary uses of spontaneous human combustion by authors other than Dickens

The matter seems to have moved almost entirely to the literary setting by the 1980s. Lee B. Croft[22] begins his article "Spontaneous Human Combustion in Literature: Some Examples of the Literary Use of Popular Mythology" with an account of a report published by United Press International in August 1982. A woman "caught fire and burned to death for no apparent reason." The UPI article included eight other instances, which, says Croft, accounts for the phenomenon of spontaneous human combustion being "firmly implanted in popular mythology."[23] He points out that, while several papers may carry the initial story, few bother to print the subsequent explanation.[24] Since, unlike science, literature is an art, an author can create a narrative to convey an explanation to the reader, rather than creating an explanation of his narrative. Thus, Croft argues, America's first professional novelist, Charles Brockden Brown (1771-1810), used spontaneous human combustion to demonstrate the evil effects of superstition in his Gothic romance *Wieland* (1798). The idea of spontaneous human combustion as a punishment for drunkenness is also used by the American novelist, Herman Melville (1819-1891), in *Redburn*. Croft states that Melville "leaves no doubt that he has Calvinist ideas in mind," using a similarity in names between his victim, Miguel Saveda, and a prominent Spanish physician and theologian, Miguel Serveto (1511-1583), who was burned at the stake for disputing Calvin's theory of the Trinity. Melville also lets the young Redburn say:

> I almost thought the burning body was a premonition of the hell of the Calvinists, and that Miguel's earthly end was a foretaste of his eternal condemnation.[25]

Similar to Dickens's use, the Russian author Nikolai Gogol (1809-1852) used spontaneous human combustion in his novel *Dead Souls* (1842) as a symbol of the corruption of a social institution, namely of serfdom. The purpose, writes Croft, is that the reader

> apprehending such a mystery as the spontaneous combustion of a diligent serf blacksmith, is supposed to say to himself, 'What a crazy world this is, where people can be bought and sold, where people can just burst into flames.'[26]

Dickens followed a similar purpose; but he was concerned that his readers hold SHC as possible which, in his view, was not out of the question. He was pointing out the danger inherent in a corrupt society, and while skeptics are likely to say he took metaphor for reality, he himself insisted that he used reality as metaphor for the working of all disease, that is – in Vrettos's words "the explosion of the private body into the public domain".[27] All of the authors used spontaneous human combustion as a literary means of influencing social justice and morality. In this, writes Croft "they hold the mysterious in common and make us wonder."[28] And of course Dickens was a great believer in the importance of wonder.

E. Muirhead Little, in the *British Medical Journal* of August 26, 1905 writes:

> If an intelligence so active and acute as that of Dickens was imposed upon[29] by the pseudo-scientific evidence in favor of this marvel (spontaneous human combustion) . . . it is small wonder that a belief in it dies hard among the wonder-loving and superstitious people who form the majority of the public.[30]

A "wonder-loving and superstitious" person would seem an unlikely description for an experienced police investigator. But the following passage was written by John Heymer, a person with just such a profession in Gwent:

> Spontaneous Human Combustion happens - there is no doubt about that. For reasons examined in this book, the Establishment chooses not to acknowledge [its] existence.[31]

Following a detailed description of the author's first encounter with SHC he writes:

> I was instantly and absolutely convinced that the scene I beheld was the aftermath of Spontaneous Human Combustion. . . . Until that day, my only knowledge of the phenomenon had been largely obtained from reading *Bleak House* by Charles Dickens, which I read with more than a little skepticism. The scene I was viewing coincided so exactly with Dickens's description of the death of Mr Krook by Spontaneous Human Combustion that it was obvious he knew what he was writing about.[32]

Heymer postulates that SHC may result from energy released across the inner membranes of cells during respiration. This would appear to be an extension of Lavoisier's[33] theory that

> respiration is nothing but a slow combustion of carbon and hydrogen, similar in all respects to that of a lamp or a lighted candle, and from this point of view, animals which breathe are really combustible substances burning and consuming themselves.[34]

Heymer sees the possibility that an excess of hydrogen and oxygen atoms coming together in a single defective mitochondrion might be sparked by the electricity generated across the membrane and result in a chain reaction throughout the body.

Jenny Randles, who has written 16 books on the paranormal, and Peter Hough, whose main research has been witchcraft, have not implausibly related this to Einstein's equation $E = MC^2$. They write:

> In his most famous equation, the physicist proved that if you do unleash the energy (E) within an atom, its power is utterly incredible. . . . If this were to occur in another form within a human body, then it is by no means unimaginable that a significant outpouring of energy could emerge from a small confined space and that this might be enough to precipitate huge levels of searing and continuing heat - in other words Spontaneous Human Combustion.[35]

This is the explanation of SHC used by the Indian novelist, Salman Rushdie (*1947), in his novel *Shame,* in which a boy is found ablaze in a parking lot:

> He burned to death, and the experts who examined his body and the scene of the incident were forced to accept what seemed impossible: namely that the boy had simply ignited of his own accord, without dousing himself in petrol or applying any external flame. *We are energy; we are light. Finding the key, stepping through that truth, the boy began to burn*[36] (my emphasis).

In the Spring of 1999, yet another article on the subject was published in *The Pharos.*[37] Dr Gamble, Professor of Orthopaedic Surgery in Stanford, California, provides a brief summary of Krook, his habits and his death. He goes on to an overview of human combustion and states that "[i]n the nineteenth century, a common belief was that people could spontaneously combust, particularly those who abused alcohol." Gamble also cites the "influential *Cyclopaedia of Practical Medicine* (1833) [which] contained a section on spontaneous combustion written by chemistry professor James Apjohn."[38] According to Gamble, the "confusion over the origin of animal heat" was one reason why the concept of human combustion did not appear unreasonable to physicians. Knowing that the body contains flammable gases and that temperature may be high during febrile diseases,

> [it] did not take a great leap of imagination to conclude that the organs could reach such a temperature that the body would burst into flames. The concept of spontaneous combustion was reinforced by preachers of the temperance movement, who embellished their sermons with the horrors of spontaneous combustion as an example of the hellish torment that awaits those who sin by drinking alcohol.[39]

Gamble ponders how Dickens came to believe so strongly in SHC and defends him to a certain degree:

> Certainly, he was too credulous . . . Literary genius that he was, Dickens did not have a scientific mind. . . . It was, however, an exciting and confusing period of transition in which no guidelines were easy to distinguish, even for men of science. Lurid sensationalists as well as serious scientists wrote about spontaneous human combustion. Furthermore, Dickens did get some bad advice from Dr Elliotson, and to this day, seemingly well-educated people are ready to believe in the weird and improbable, including the healing power of crystals, invasion by space aliens, monsters, angels, and even spontaneous human combustion.[40]

One last article remains to be discussed, an article which takes the whole matter in an entirely different direction. Sheila Shaw, professor of English at Wheaton College, draws a connection between these supposed burnings and menopause, pointing out that the victims were usually old women. She, too, cites the well-known stories of Countess Bandi, Mary Clues, and Grace Pitt. All of these accounts include a description of the remains and Shaw is struck by the images of dismemberment, claiming that the "arrangement" of Cornelia Bandi's remains was "sexually suggestive, since her head (the brain of which . . . had been consumed) lay between the legs."[41] One must ask where, considering that the torso was incinerated and the remains were reportedly about four feet from the bed, Shaw might expect the head of a person who died in an upright position to land? And a fire which consumed bone, muscle and viscera would not surprisingly have destroyed brain tissue. It would appear that Shaw has read in stereotypical biases where none need be assumed. She writes:

> Not to be underestimated in this scenario is the role played by . . . a medical profession that increasingly violated women's bodies on the dissecting tables and in anatomical textbooks, regarding them important only as bearers of live babies.[42]

Shaw overlooks the fact that the medical profession had performed dissections even in the Middle Ages, and that the limited supply of cadavers (see Chapter 7) precluded there being much choice in gender. The woman's child-bearing function was at one and the same time her main role in survival of the species and the greatest danger to her personal health and well-being. Advances in obstetrics and gynecology based at least in part on knowledge gained in dissections, coupled with sterile techniques, were largely the means of reducing the death rates of both mother and child. Moreover, as Shaw also discusses, comparative anatomy - like most specialized areas - was relatively new and of growing importance. The late twentieth century could provide "virtual dissection laboratories" - but earlier doctors needed cadavers - of both sexes. It is curious that Shaw appears to be very ambivalent about the facts and to have problems remaining objective. She cites pornographic verse as "evidence" of the sexual bias in SHC, claiming that both "highlight an interest in sectioning the female body."[43]

Shaw goes on to say:

> This much is clear: whoever wrote the various examples of female bodies and spontaneous combustion was supported by a tradition that sanctioned a pathological vision of elderly women as dismembered, eviscerated, and torched. Their reproductive capacity gone, too old to be objects of male desire, and with no outlet for innate carnal appetites, they implode. The fire that consumes them is a time-honored mode of punishment, as any sixteenth-century woman accused of witchcraft and burned alive at the stake might have told us.[44]

Having read more than just the classical and best-known cases, and remembering that Brown's, Melville's, Gogol's, Dickens's and Twain's[45] victims were all males (Melville's even paralleling a *man* who was burned at the stake - albeit for heresy, not witchcraft), the validity of Shaw's statement may be questioned.[46]

Personal contact with John Heymer revealed that he is still convinced that the phenomenon exists, even though it cannot yet be explained. He points out the impossibility of conducting conclusive experiments, which cannot be *spontaneous*. Also, the victim must be alive at the time and who would volunteer, even if the mechanism were clear? The likelihood that such a case will happen in the presence of a scientist is small, so absolute proof – or absolute disproof – may never be obtained.

For Dickens, as for other novelists, SHC existed. The phenomenon provided a metaphor which could not have been more horrifying or more apt. His statement in the Preface that he had "dwelt on the romantic side of familiar things" does not qualify his use of the phenomenon. The "familiar things" in the novel include smallpox, poverty, pollution, bogus charity, etc. SHC, while the subject of several reports, hardly had the degree of familiarity of these social problems. Since, as discussed, the matter was of interest in medical jurisprudence, Dickens's use of SHC can also be taken as further evidence of his interest in the medical matters of his day. Whether we choose to believe or disbelieve, the episode remains a compelling piece of writing. As the physiologist, John West, writes:

> For the physiologist of today, the remarkable thing is that there was so much earnest discussion of the preposterous notion that spontaneous combustion could occur. . . . Whether it is physiologically possible or not (and the answer is not) is immaterial to its dramatic contribution to *Bleak House*.[47]

[1] Trevor Blount. "Dickens and Mr Krook's Spontaneous Combustion" *DSA*, I 1970, 182-211; here 186.
[2] Harrison (1977), 22/23.
[3] Claude-Nicholas Lecat, 1700-1768, French surgeon.
[4] See for example *Letters*, 7:28-31; Collins, *Heritage* (1971), 275; Ackroyd (1990), 662.
[5] Arnold (1995), 21.
[6] *Letters*, 7:28-31.
[7] *Letters*, 7. Elliotson, of course, was himself considered something of a medical maverick which may explain *why* Dickens didn't mention him.
[8] Harrison (1977), 46/47.
[9] This term may well be a typographical error in the text. Logically, the word should be "empyresmus", although even that was apparently coined by Ogston.
[10] *BMJ* March 19, 1870, 294.
[11] Gould and Pyle (1896), 426-429.
[12] Harrison (1977), 154.
[13] Paris and Fonblanque (1823), 412.
[14] who was, however, not identified.
[15] Paris and Fonblanque (1823), 412.
[16] François Emanuel Fodéré, 1764-1835; Charles Chrétien Henri Marc, 1771-1841.
[17] Paris and Fonblanque (1823),414.
[18] *Ibid*, 415.
[19] DiMaio and DiMaio (1989), 341.
[20] Knight (1996), 316.
[21] Phillips (2003), 22 23.
[22] Croft (1989), 335.
[23] *The Arizona Republic*, 6. August 1982, p A-4. Cited in Croft (1989), 335.
[24] This conveniently ignores obvious fact that even those who, in all open-mindedness, have come to believe in the phenomenon *can't* explain it – yet, anyway.
[25] Herman Melville, *Redburn: His First Voyage*. Evanston. Northwestern University Press and Newberry Library, 1969, 244. Cited in Croft (1989), 342.
[26] Nikolai Gogol, *Dead Souls*, trans Andrew R. MacAndrew. New York, 1961, 59-60. Cited in Croft (1989), 344.
[27] Vrettos (1995), 5.
[28] *Ibid*, 347.
[29] The phrase "imposed upon" is curious; Dickens was convinced – willingly it appears – by what he considered conclusive evidence. Obviously Little did not share Dickens's belief.
[30] Cited in Arnold., 61.
[31] This raises a curious echo of Dickens's letter to Elliotson cited above.
[32] Heymer (1996), 4.
[33] Antoine-Laurent Lavoisier, (1743-1794), French pioneer in chemistry.
[34] Lavoisier. *Premier Mémoire sur la Respiration des Animaux* (1789) in: West (1994), 126.
[35] Randles and Hough (1996).
[36] This notice was submitted to the *Dickensian* 91 (1995) by Mrs Vikki Ryhiner of Bern.
[37] Gamble (1999), 11.
[38] *Ibid*, 12.
[39] *Ibid*, 13.
[40] *Ibid*, 15. Gamble cites here an article by M. Benecke: "Spontaneous human combustion: Thoughts of a forensic biologist." *Skeptical Inquirer*, 1998; 22 (2):47-51.
[41] Shaw, (1995).

[42] *Ibid*, 18.
[43] *Ibid*, 9.
[44] *Ibid*, 18.
[45] Jimmy Finn in *Life on the Mississppi*.
[46] Shaw's explanation here would undoubtedly be "that men also combust seems to be, mostly, a nineteenth-century afterthought, for tales of such phenomena began to spread only after the publication of Lair's essay in 1800." Several male victims were, however, reported prior to that time.
[47] West (1994), 125, 128.

CONCLUSION

In 1955, Lord Brain said that Dickens gave "detailed and accurate descriptions of the disorders from which his characters suffered" and that he "looked on disease with the observing eye of the expert clinician and . . . often gives us accounts which would do credit to a trained physician." My aim in writing this dissertation has been to subject these statements to critical examination and create a basis on which they could be proved or rejected. My research has brought very strong evidence in support of Brain's statement. A large variety of disorders is to be found. Literary criticism has often either not recognized the state or misinterpreted it, depending apparently on the degree to which the disease/disorder is known among laymen and the metaphoric or symbolic importance which could be attributed to it.

A medical-historical reading of the texts reveals that Dickens's observations and descriptions of things medical are realistic and accurate. This has been demonstrated by comparing his descriptions with those in medical journals and texts available in his day. Medical publications up to the present have been consulted to examine whether medical progress has brought contradictory knowledge to light. Not only is this *not* the case, but medical writers have identified several clinical states in reading Dickens's descriptions which had not been medically identified at the time he was writing.

What makes Dickens unique among Victorian writers is not only his use but also the variety of identifiable diseases he describes. Twenty-four diseases/disorders can be found, many of them in secondary characters and without any apparent uniform symbolic use. Interesting is that the details are just as realistic in minor and major diseases or disabilities. Three major diseases are used in several novels and each time in a form both suited to the plot and the character yet adhering to medical reality. Epilepsy is used in the traditional trope of manifest evil of the individual, but also sociocritically as manifest evil of an institution; stroke in several of its forms is revealed as retribution for bad parenting; tuberculosis is used to stir public awareness of problems of poverty, health and sanitation.

Like tuberculosis, smallpox, provision for orphaned or abandoned children, sanitation and housing, metropolitan burial grounds and substance abuse are issues of public health in Victorian England to be found in Dickens's novels. The political currency of his writing can be traced in both medical and lay press of the time. Among such issues, the hitherto unnoticed coincidence of smallpox in *Bleak House* with the reading of the Compulsory Vaccination Bill emphasises the topicality of Dickens's writings.

Descriptions of folk medicine and popular remedies are to be found in Dickens's works. It is noted that several of these remedies were used by Dickens himself and others were included in popular home remedy books of the late-eighteenth and nineteenth centuries.

Spontaneous Human Combustion, long considered a myth, but one in which Dickens believed, was fiercely debated in the nineteenth century and in the late twentieth as well. It is found that there are still skeptics and believers: since scientific proof cannot be obtained – the word "spontaneous" rules out any real possibility of proof or disproof - this chapter ends with a question mark.

Overall, however, no question remains concerning the variety or accuracy of medical episodes in Dickens's works. The study has augmented our appreciation of Dickens's powers of both observation and description and has also provided new insight into some of his motives for and aspects of his writings which have as yet been neglected. It locates the medical episodes within Dickens's vast writings, thus facilitating the investigation of language in the fictional description of disease, the impact of disease prevalence on the literature of a given age, the importance of illness in the human experience from a realistic and a metaphorical perspective, as well as other related topics.

Bibliography

Works by Dickens

Pickwick Papers. Oxford World's Classics, 1988, James Kinsley, ed.
Oliver Twist. Oxford, Clarendon Press, 1974. Kathleen Tillotson, ed.
Nicholas Nickleby. Oxford, Oxford University Press, 1982.
The Old Curiosity Shop. Oxford, Clarendon 1997, Elizabeth Brennan, ed.
Barnaby Rudge. London, Penguin, 1986. Gordon Spence, ed.
Martin Chuzzlewit. Oxford, Clarendon, 1982. Margaret Cardwell, ed.
Dombey and Son. Oxford World's Classics, 1996. Alan Horsman, ed.
David Copperfield. Oxford, Clarendon, 1981. Nina Burgess, ed.
Dr Marigold's Prescriptions. The New York Publishing Company, date unknown.
Bleak House. London. Penguin, 1994.
Hard Times. London. Penguin, 1983. David Craig, ed.
Little Dorrit. Oxford, Clarendon, 1979. Harvey Peter Sucksmith, ed.
A Tale of Two Cities. London, Penguin, 1988. George Woodcock, ed.
Great Expectation.s New York, Norton, 1999. Edgar Rosenberg, ed.
Our Mutual Friend. London, Penguin, 1987. Stephen Gill, ed.
Mystery of Edwin Drood. Oxford, Clarendon, 1972. Margaret Cardwell, ed.
The Christmas Books, London, Penguin, reprint 1984. Michael Slater, ed.
"A Christmas Carol" and "The Chimes"
Sketches by Boz in *Dickens' Journalism*, 1. London, Phoenix. Michael Slater, ed.
"Review: *Narrative of the Expedition sent by her Majesty's Government to the river Niger in 1841..." The Examiner*, 19 August 1848. in: *Dickens' Journalism.* 2, London, Dent. Michael Slater, ed.
Uncommercial Traveller in *Dickens' Journalism*, 4. London, Dent. Michael Slater, ed.
American Notes. London. Penguin, 1987. John Whitley and Arnold Goldman, eds.
The Letters of Charles Dickens. Oxford. The Pilgrim Edition, Madeline House, et al. eds.
Household Words. London, Bradbury and Evans.
All the Year Round. London, Chapman and Hall.
Charles Dickens: *Uncollected Writings from Household Words 1850-1859.* Harry Stone, Ed. Bloomington & London, Indiana University Press, 1968.
The Speeches of Charles Dickens. K.J. Fielding, ed. Hemel Hempstead, Harvester Wheatsheaf, 1988.

Primary Medical Sources
Aitkin, William. *The Practice of Medicine.* London, Charles Griffin and Company, 1866.
Buchan, William. *Domestic Medicine.* Edition V. Exeter, J.B. Williams, 1828.
DiMaio and DiMaio, *Forensic Pathology*, New York, Elsevier 1989.
Down, J. Langdon (ed). *Alcohol. Its Use and Abuse.* Health Primers. London, 1878.

Enzyklopaedisches Wörterbuch der medicinischen Wissenschaften. D.W.H. Busch et al., eds. Berlin, Boike 1828-42.

Gould, George M. and Pyle, Walter L. *Anomalies and Curiosities of Medicine.* New York, Bell, 1896.

Harrison's Principles of Internal Medicine, 9th ed. Kurt J. Isselbacher, et al. eds. London. McGraw Hill, 1980.

Hassall, A.H. *Food and its Adulterations.* Comprising the Report of the Analytical Sanitary Commission of *The Lancet* for the years 1851 to 1854, inclusive. London, 1855.

Knight, Bernard. *Forensic Pathology,* second edition, London, Arnold, 1996.

Lennox, William Gordon. *Epilepsy and Related Disorders.* Boston, Little, Brown. 1960.

Miller, James. *Principles of Surgery.* London, Longman, 1850.

Merck Manual, Robert Berkow, M.D., ed., 13th Edition. Rahway, New Jersey, 1977.

Paris, J.A. and Fonblanque, J.M. *Medical Jurisprudence in 3 Volumes.* London, W. Phillips, 1823.

Pettigrew, Thomas Joseph. *On Superstition connected with the History and Practice of Medicine and Surgery.* London, J. Churchill, 1844.

Pfaltz, E.R. and Alford, B.R., eds. *Controversial Aspects of Ménière's Disease.* Stuttgart and New York, Thieme Verlag, 1986.

Real-Encyclopädie der gesammten Heilkunde. 3. Auflage. Prof. Dr Albert Wulenburg, Hrsg. Vienna and Leipzig, Urban & Schwarzenberg, 1894.

Ried, S., Schüler, G. *Epilepsie. Vom Anfall bis zur Zusammenarbeit.* Berlin, Blackwell-Wiss.-Verl. 1997.

Shorvon, Simon et al., eds. *The Treatment of Epilepsy,* Oxford , Blackwell Science, 1996.

Tidy, Charles Meymott. *Legal Medicine,* I and II. London, William Wood, 1882.

Tissot, S.A.D. *Abhandlung von der Epilepsie oder fallenden Sucht.* Translation to German by J.S. Krünißβ, Berlin, Hande & Spener, 1771.

Wolf, Peter, ed. *Epileptic Seizures and Syndromes with some of their theoretical implications.* London. John Libbey & Co., Ltd., 1994.

Other Literary and Critical Sources

[anonymous] "Mr Wakley's Petition Against the Anatomy Law". *The Lancet,* 1829:306-9

Ackroyd, Peter. *Charles Dickens.* London, Sinclair-Stevenson, 1990.

Adams, Norman. *Dead and Buried: the horrible history of bodysnatching.* Aberdeen, Impulse, 1972.

Adrian, Arthur A. *Dickens and the Parent-Child Relationship.* Athens (Ohio) and London. Ohio University Press, 1984.

Alison, William P. *Reply to Dr Chalmers' Objections to an Improvement of the Legal Provision for the Poor in Scotland.* Edinburgh, William Blackwood, 1841.

Amalric, Jean-Claude, ed. *Studies in the later Dickens.* Montpellier, Univ. Paul Valéry. 1973.

Altick, Richard. *The Presence of the Present. Topics of the Day in the Victorian Novel.* Columbus, Ohio State University Press, 1991.

Altman, Roy D. "Paget's Disease of Bone". In Kiple (1993), 911-914.

Andrews, Malcolm. Introduction to *The Old Curiosity Shop*. London, Penguin English Library, 1972.

Andrews, Malcolm. "Dickens and the medical profession." *The New Zealand Medical Journal,* 1985:810-13.

Arnold, Larry E. *Ablaze! The Mysterious Fires of Spontaneous Human Combustion*. New York, Evans, 1995.

Bailey, James Blake. *The Diary of a Resurrectionist*. London, S. Sonnenschein & Co., 1896.

Bailin, Miriam. *The Sickroom in Victorian Fiction. The Art of Being Ill*. Cambridge, Cambridge University Press, 1994.

Baldwin, Peter. *Contagion and the State in Europe*. Cambridge, Cambridge University Press, 1999.

Barry, Jonathan and Colin Jones. *Medicine and Charity Before the Welfare State*. London, Routledge, 1991.

Bateman, David: "Dickens: an alternative diagnosis." Letter to *The Lancet* 359, 2002:1253.

Berridge, Virginia. "Victorian Opium-Eating: Responses to opiate use in nineteenth-century England". *Victorian Studies* 21, 1978:437-61.

Berridge, Virginia. "The Era of Public Health. 1848-1918. in: Webster, 63-86.

Berridge, Virginia. *Opium and the people: opiate use and drug control policy in the nineteenth and early twentieth century England.* London, Free Association, 1999.

Bethel, Robert.: "The Longer I Live, the more I doubt the Doctors." *St. Mary's Hospital Gazette* 76, 1970:12-13 and 25.

Bettesworth, A. *Seasonable Considerations on the Indecent and Dangerous Custom of Burying in Churches and Church-Yards with remarkable Observations Historical and Philosophical Proving that the Custom is not only Contrary to the Practice of the Antients, but fatal, in Case of Infection.* Sandwich, 1721.

Bibliographisches Lexikon der hervorragenden Ärzte aller Zeiten und Völker. Prof. F. Hűbotter (Berlin) and Prof. H. Vierordt (Tűbingen) editors. Berlin/Vienna, 1908.

Blount, Trevor. "Dickens and Mr Krook's Spontaneous Combustion". *Dickens Studies Annual* (1970) I:183-211.

Bowen, John. *The Other Dickens. Pickwick to Chuzzlewit.* Oxford, Oxford University Press, 2000.

Bowen, W.H. *Charles Dickens and His Family. A Sympathetic Study*. Cambridge. W. Heffer & Sons, Ltd., 1956.

Bowlby, John. *A Secure Base*. Parent-Child Attachment and Healthy Human Development. London, Routledge, 1988.

Brain, R. "Dickensian Diagnoses": in *Some Reflections on Genius*. London, Pitman, 1955.

Brennan, Elizabeth M. Introduction to *The Old Curiosity Shop*. Oxford, Clarendon Press, 1997

Briggs, Asa. *Collected Essays*. Brighton, Harvester, 1985.

Brontë, Charlotte. *Shirley*. Andrew and Judith Hook, eds. London, Penguin , 1974.

Brogunier, Joseph. "The Funeral Pyre and Human Decency: The Fate of Chancery in *Bleak House*." *The Dickensian* 61, 1965:57-62.

Browning, L.D. "mesmerism" in Schlicke (1999), 375.
Bynum, W.F. and Porter, Roy, eds. *Companion Encyclopedia of the History of Medicine.* London and New York, Routledge, 1993.
Bynum, W.F. and Porter, Roy, eds. *Medical Fringe and Medical Orthodoxy 1750-1850.* London. Croom Helm, 1987.
Bynum, W.F. *Science and the Practice of medicine in the Nineteenth Century.* Cambridge. Cambridge University Press, 1994.
Callahan, Charles W. Jr. "Tiny Tim: The Child with a Crippling Fatal Illness". *The Dickensian* 89, 1993:214-17.
Carter, A.J.: "A Christmas Carol. Charles Dickens and the birth of orthopaedics." *Journal of the Royal Society of Medicine* 86, 1993:45-48
Carter, Geoffrey. "Sexuality and the Victorian Artist": Dickens and Swinburne. In: Cox (1984), 141-160.
Carter, Henry. *The English Temperance Movement. A Study in Objectives.* London, Epworth Press, 1933.
Cartwright, Frederick F. *A Social History of Medicine.* London and New York, Longman, 1977.
Castiglioni, Arturo. *A History of Medicine*. New York, Aronson, 1975.
Chesney, Russell. "Bah! Humbug!" *The American Journal of the Diseases of Children* 47, 1993:818.
Chittick, Kathryn. *Dickens and the 1830s.* Cambridge, Cambridge University Press, 1990.
Collings, E. *National Magazine and Monthly Critic* , December 1837. Reprinted in *The Dickensian I-II, 9-13.*
Collins, Philip. *Dickens and Education*. London, Macmillan, 1965.
Collins, Philip. *A Critical Commentary on Dickens's Bleak House.* London, Macmillan, 1971.
Collins, Philip. *Dickens. The Critical Heritage.* London, Macmillan, 1971.
Collins, Philip. "How many men was Dickens the novelist?" in Amalric, 1973.
Collins, Philip. "Physicians in Victorian Fiction." In: *Art and Society in the Victorian Novel.* Ed. Colin Gibson. London, Macmillan, 1989.
Connor, Stephen. *Charles Dickens.* London, Longman, 1996.
Cooter, Roger. *The Cultural Meaning of Popular Science.* Cambridge, Cambridge University Press, 1984.
Cosnett, J.E. "Charles Dickens: Observer of Sleep and Its Disorders." *Sleep* 15(3), 1992:264-267.
Cosnett, J.E. "Dickens and doctors: vignettes of Victorian medicine." *British Medical Journal* 305, 1992:1542.
Cosnett, J.E. "Charles Dickens and Epilepsy". *Epilepsia.* 53(4), 1994:903-905.
Cosnett, J.E. "Charles Dickens and Sleep Disorders." *The Dickensian*. 93, 1997:200-204.
Cosnett, J.E. Letter to the Editor, *The Dickensian* 94, 1998:131.
Cosnett, J.E. Letter to the Editor. *Addiction* 94 (23), 1999:1891-92.
Cosnett, J.E. "Charles Dickens - Syndrome Spotter. A Review of some Morbid Observations." *The Dickensian* 2003:22-31.

Cox, Arthur J. “Magnetic Sympathy in *The Mystery of Edwin Drood.*” *The Dickensian* 2000:127-150; and 209-242.

Cox, Don Richard, Ed. *Sexuality and Victorian Literature.* Knoxville, University of Tennessee Press, 1984.

Croft, Lee B. “Spontaneous Human Combustion in Literature: Some examples of the literary use of popular mythology.” *CLA Journal College Language Association* 32, 1989:335-347.

Crowther, M. Anne. “health, illness and disability” in: Schlicke (1999), 266-268.

Curl, James Stevens. *The Victorian Celebration of Death.* London, Abbot, David and Charles, 1972.

DaCosta, John Chalmers. *Dickens's Doctors.* Philadelphia, Philobiblon Club, 1905.

Darwin, B. “Dickens's Doctors,” *British Medical Journal* 1952:1039-40.

DeQuincey, Thomas. *Confessions of an English Opium Eater.* London. George Routledge Sons, [new edition], 1867.

Dickens, David and Jacoby, Norman. “Charles Dickens's Travelling Medicine Chest.” *The Dickensian* 92, 1997:19-24.

Dudgeon, Piers. *Dickens' London. An Imaginative Vision.* London, Headline, 1987.

Duncan, B.M.: “Chloroform for Mrs Dickens.” *The History of Anaesthesia Society Proceedings* 1989:31-33.

Duncan-Jones, E.E. “Mrs Harris & Deputy.” *The Dickensian* 1971:119.

Dunn, Frederick. “Malaria” in Kiple (1993), 855-872.

Durey, M.J. “Bodysnatchers and Benthamites. The Implications of the Dead Body Bill for the London Schools of Anatomy, 1820-1842.” *The London Journal. A Review of Metropolitan Society Past and Present* 1, 1976:200-25.

Eagleton, Terry. “*Doctor Glas:* haunting reflections.” *The Lancet* 360, 2002:2092.

Eco, Umberto. *Derrick oder die Leidenschaft für das Mittelmaß.* Streichholzbriefe 1990-2000. Translated by Burkhart Kroebar. Munich, Hauser, 2000.

Eliot, George. *The Mill on the Floss* (1860). Sally Shuttleworth, ed. London, Routledge, 1991.

Eliot, George. *Middlemarch.* Rosemary Ashton, ed. London, Penguin, 1994.

Engel, Monroe. *The Maturity of Dickens.* Cambridge/MA, Harvard University Press, 1959.

Epstein Nord, Deborah. *Walking the Victorian Streets. Women, Representation and the City.* Ithaca and London, Cornell University Press, 1995.

“J.W.F.” “Bob Sawyer and Ben Allen vindicated by a doctor”. *The Dickensian* 1915-16, 188-190

Fasick, Laura. “Dickens and the Diseased Body in *Bleak House.*” *Dickens Studies Annual* 24, 1996:134-151.

Fay, Peter Ward. *The Opium War, 1840-42.* Chapel Hill, University of North Carolina Press, 1975.

Feder, Lillian. *Madness in Literature.* Princeton, Princeton University Press, 1980.

Fido, Martin. *Bodysnatchers. A History of the Resurrectionists. 1742-1832.* London, Hamlyn, 1988.

Fiedler, Leslie. “Images of the nurse in fiction and popular culture.” *Literature and Medicine* 2, 1985:78-90.

Fielding, Henry. *Tom Jones*. R.C.P. Mutter, ed,. London, Penguin, 1985.

Fielding, K.J. "Dickens's work with Miss Coutts: I. Nova Scotia Gardens and What Grew There." *The Dickensian* 61, 1965:112-19.

Fielding, K.J. "Dickens's work with Miss Coutts: II. Casby and the Westminster Landlords." *Ibid:*155-160.

Fielding, K.J. "*Bleak House* and Dickens' Originals. The Romantic Side of Familiar Things." *Dickens Studies Annual,* 24, 1996:119-134.

Fildes, Valerie. *Breasts, Bottles and Babies. A History of Infant Feeding.* Edinburgh, University of Edinburgh Press, 1986.

Finnegan, Frances. *Poverty and Prostitution: a study of Victorian prostitutes in York.*
Cambridge, Cambridge University Press, 1979.

Forster, John. *The Life of Charles Dickens.* London, Chapman & Hall, 1899.

Foucault, Michel. *Die Geburt der Klinik* (German: Walter Seitter). Frankfurt, Fischer Taschenbuch Verlag, 1996.

Fowler, R. "Polyphony and Problematic in *Hard Times.*" In: Connor, Steven, ed. *Charles Dickens.* London, Longman, 1996, 107-8.

Freedman, A.L. "Dickens, Dombey and Diagnostics." *Annals of Internal Medicine* 84, 1984:102:271.

Furst, Lilian R. *Between Doctors and Patient. The changing balance of power.* Charlottesville, University Press of Virginia, 1998.

Gamble, James. "Charles Dickens: His quaint little "person of the house," and the English Disease. *The Pharos* 1996:24-28.

Gamble, James. "Charles Dickens gets a Lesson in Sensitivity." *The Pharos*, 1998:8-12.

Gamble, James. "Death by spontaneous combustion: Charles Dickens and the strange case of Mr Krook." *The Pharos,* 1999:11-15.

Gaskell, E. "Dickens and Medicine". London, The Wellcome Institute, 1970.

Gaskell, Elizabeth. *Mary Barton. A Tale of Manchester Life.*(1848) London, Penguin Classics, 1996.

Gaskell, Elizabeth. *Cranford* (1853). London, Penguin Popular Classics, 1994.

Gates, Barbara T.: *Victorian Suicide. Mad Crimes and Sad Histories.* Princeton University Press, Princeton, 1988.

Gay, Peter. *Savage Reprisals. Bleak House, Madame Bovary, Buddenbrooks.* New York and London, W.W. Norton & Company, 2002.

Geisler, L.S.: "Das Pickwick-Syndrom" *Deutsche Medizinische Wochenschrift* 5, 1971:212-16.

Gelfert, Hans-Dieter. *Die Symbolik im Romanwerk von Charles Dickens.* Stuttgart, Berlin, Köln, Mainz, Verlag W. Kohlhammmer, 1974.

Geppert, Hans Vilmar. *Der realistische Weg. Formen pragmatischen Erzählens bei Balzac, Dickens, Hardy, Keller, Raabe und anderen Autoren des 19. Jahrhunderts.* Tübingen, Max Niemeyer Verlag, 1994.

Gilman, Sander L. *Difference and Pathology: Stereotypes of sexuality, race and madness.* Ithaca and London, Cornell University Press, 1985.

Gilman, Sander L. *Disease and Representation. Images of Illness from Madness to AIDS.* Ithaca and London, Cornell University Press, 1988.
Gilman, Sander L. *Health and Illness. Images of Difference.* London, Reaktion Books, 1995
Gilmour, Robin. *The Victorian Period.* London, Longman, 1993.
Glover, Dr Robert M. "The Philosopy of Medicine". *The Lancet*, January 11, 1851, 35-38.
Goetsch, Paul. *Dickens.* Munich, Artemis, 1986.
Graham, John: *Lavater's Essays on Physiognomy. A Study in the History of Ideas.* Bern, Peter Lang, 1979.
Grant, Dorothy. "History of the Wet Nurse." *The Medical Post (Canada)* February 22, 2000, 21.
Greyson, Bruce. "Dissociation in people who have near-death experiences: out of their bodies or out of their minds?" *The Lancet* 356, 2000:460-3.
Grove, Thelma. "Barnaby Rudge" A Case Study in Autism." *The Dickensian* 83, 1987:139-148.
Guida, Fred. *A Christmas Carol and Its Adaptations. A Critical Examination of Dickens's Story and Its Productions on Screen and Television.* McFarland, London, 2000.
Gurney, Michael. "Disease as Device: The Role of Smallpox in *Bleak House*". *Literature and Medicine* 9, 1990:79-82.
Haeser, Heinrich, Hsgr. *Geschichte der Medicin und der epidemischen Krankheiten.* Jena, Gustav Fischer, 1882.
Hamlin, Christopher. *Public Health and Social Justice in the Age of Chadwick: Britain, 1800-1854.* Cambridge and NY, Cambridge U Press, 1998.
Hardwick, Michael and Mollie. *The Charles Dickens Encyclopedia.* Reading, Osprey, 1973.
Hardy, Anne. "St. Anthony's Fire" in Kiple (1993), 989-990.
Hardy, Anne. *The Epidemic Streets: infectious disease and the rise of preventive medicine, 1856-1900.* Oxford, Clarendon Press, 1993.
Hardy, Anne. *Health and Medicine in Britain since 1860.* Houndsmills and New York. Palgrave, 2001
Harrison, J.F.C. "Early Victorian Radicals and the Medical Fringe." In: Bynum and Porter (1987), 216-233.
Harrison, Michael. *Fire from Heaven. A Study of Spontaneous Combustion in Human Beings.* Revised ed. London & Sydney, Pan Books, 1977.
Hartley, Lucy. *Physiognomy and the Meaning of Expression in Nineteenth-Century Culture.* Cambridge, Cambridge University Press, 2001
Herrmann, M. *Schlafapnoe als Krankheitskonstrukt: Die Mechanisierung und Medikalisierung des Schlafes.* Frankfurt, Campus-Verlag, 1997.
Heymer, John E. *The Entrancing Flame. The Facts of Spontaneous Human Combustion.* London, Little, Brown & Co., 1996.
Higgenbottham, Ann R. "Sin of the Age: Infanticide and Illegitimacy in Victorian London." *Victorian Studies* 32, 1989:319-337.
Hill, T.W. "Notes on *The Old Curiosity Shop*" *The Dickensian* 64, 1953:137-142.
Hillis Miller, J. *Charles Dickens. The World of his Novels.* Cambridge MA, Harvard University Press, 1958.

Hobsbaum, Philip. *A Reader's Guide to Charles Dickens*. London, Thames + Hudson, 1972.
Hochman, Baruch and Ilja Wachs. *Dickens. The Orphan Condition*. Madison, Fairleigh Dickinson University Press, 1999.
Howell, W.B., MD. "Some Humble Workers in the Cause of Anatomy a Hundred Years Ago." *Annals of Medical History* 8, 1926:2-30.
Iser, Wolfgang. *The Implied Reader*. Baltimore, Johns Hopkins University, 1990.
Jacoby, N.M.: "Charles Dickens' Asthma" *Journal of Medical Biography* (1995) 3:34-42.
Jacoby, N.M.: "Krook's Dyslexia." *The Dickensian* 91, 1995:102-107.
Johnson, Edgar. *Charles Dickens. His Tragedy and Triumph.* New York, Simon & Schuster, 1952.
Jones, Pamela. *Shepherd's Bush: the Dickens Connection.* London, Shepherd's Bush Local Historical Society, 1992.
Jones, Paul G.: "Dickens' Literary Children." *The Australian Paediatrics Journal* 8, 1972:233-245.
Judd, Catherine. "Nine Oils or the Balm of Bilead. Nursing and Social Healing in *Hard Times*." The Dickens Project, University of California 1990, 191-97.
Kaplan, Fred. *Dickens and Mesmerism. The Hidden Springs of Fiction*. Princeton, Princeton University, 1975.
Kaplan, Fred. *Dickens*. New York, William Morrow & Co., 1988.
Kinder, Sue. "A mesmerizing tale." *The Lancet*, 360, 2002:1992-3.
Kiple, Kenneth F. ed. *Cambridge World History of Human Diseases*. Cambridge, Cambridge University Press, 1993.
Kryger, M.H. "Sleep Apnea: From the Needles of Dionysius to Continuous Positive Airway Pressure." *Archives of Internal Medicine*, 143, 1983:2301-2303.
Kryger, M.H. "Fat, Sleep and Charles Dickens." *Clinics in Chest Medicine* 6, 1985:555-563.
Lavie, P. "Nothing New Under the Moon - Historical Accounts of Sleep Apnea Syndrome." *Archives of. Internal Medicine* 144, 1984:2025-28.
Layton, T.B. "Dickens's Medical Students," *Guy's Hospital Gazette*, 50,1936:553-562.
Leavis, F.R. and Q.D. *Dickens the Novelist*. London 1970; Penguin reprint, 1994.
Lerner, Laurence. *Angels and Absences. Child Deaths in the Nineteenth Century*. Nashville, Vanderbilt University Press, 1997.
LeSage, Alain-René. *Die Geschichte des Gil Blas von Santillana.* (Translated by Fink) Munich, Winkler, 1981.
Leven, Karl-Heinz. "Krankheiten – historische Deutung versus retrospektive Diagnose." In: Paul and Schlich (1998), 153-185.
Lewis, D.W. "What was wrong with Tiny Tim?" *American Journal of the Diseases of Children* 146, 1992:1403-1407.
Lohrli, Anne. *Household Words. Table of Contents, List of Contributors and their Contributions*. Toronto, University of Toronto Press, 1973.
London, S.J. "The Whimsey Syndrome." *Archives of .Internal Medicine* 122, 1968:448-52.
Loudon, Irvine. *Death in Childbirth.* Oxford, Clarendon Press, 1992.
Loudon, Irvine. *Western Medicine. An Illustrated History.* Oxford, Oxford University Press, 1997.

Mackenzie, William. *An Appeal to the Public and to the Legislature on the necessity of affording Dead Bodies to the Schools of Anatomy by Legislative Enactment.* Glasgow, 1824.

Maidlow, W.H. "A Note on Charles Dickens and the Doctors." *St. Bartholomew's Hospital Journal*, 1917:52.

Markel, Howard. "Charles Dickens and the Art of Medicine." *Annals of Internal Medicine*, 1984:101, 408-411.

Markel, Howard. "In Defense of the Pickwickian Syndrome." *Henry Ford Hospital Medical Journal* 33, 1985:24-6.

Markel, Howard. Letter to the Editor, *The Dickensian* 76, 1982:120-1.

Marshall, Tim. "Bodies for Dissection. The 1832 Anatomy Act." *The N.A.N.I.M.E. Journal* 13, 1999:17-21.

McHugh, Paul. *Prostitution and Victorian Social Reform.* London, Croom Helm, 1980.

McManus, I.C.: "Charles Dickens: a neglected diagnosis." *The Lancet* 358, 2001:2158-61.

McPhail, Alexander. "The After-math of Body-snatching: A Plea for Anatomy." *St. Bartholomew's Hospital Journal.* 1916:28-34.

Milligan, Barry. *Pleasures and Pains: Opium and the Orient in nineteenth-century British Culture.* Charlottesville, University Press of Virginia, 1995.

Nelson, Roxanne. "Neonatal and childhood stroke remain underdiagnosed." *The Lancet* 360, 2002:1306.

Nelson, Roxanne. "The Case of Tiny Tim." *The Washington Post.* December 24, 2002, HE01.

O'Hara, Dwight; "Dr Charles Dickens.".*New England Journal of Medicine.* 1939:1082-86.

Oppenheim, Janet. *Shattered Nerves: doctors, patients and depression in Victorian England.* New York, Oxford University Press, 1991.

Oppenlander, Ella Ann. *Dickens's All the Year Round. Descriptive Index and Contributor List.* Troy, The Whitston Publishing Company, 1984.

Orton, Diane. *Made of Gold. A Biography of Angela Burdett Coutts.* London, Hamish Hamilton, 1980.

Pahor, Ahmes L. "Charles Dickens and the Ear, Nose and Throat." *Archives of Otolaryngology* 105, 1979:1-5.

Paul, Norbert and Schlich, Thomas, ed. *Medizingeschichte: Aufgaben, Probleme, Perspektiven.* Frankfurt and New York, Campus Verlag, 1998.

Pederson, Winnifred J. "Jo in *Bleak House.*" *The Dickensian* 60, 1964:162- 167.

Pellegrini, Ernestina. *Necropoli Immaginarie. Le Rappresentazioni della Morte in Balzac, Flaubert, Zola, Dickens, Dostoevskij e Tolstoj.* Le Lettere, Firenze, 1996.

Peterson, Douglas. "What was wrong with Tiny Tim?" *The American Journal of the Diseases of Children* 47, 1993:818-9.

Peterson, M. Jeanne. *The Medical Profession in Mid-Victorian London.* Berkeley, University of California Press, 1978.

Phillips, Michelle. "History of the Human Candle." *The Medical Post (Canada).* January 28, 2003, 22-23.

Piller, Gordon. "John Hughes Bennett. His Life and the Identification of Leukaemia." *Proceedings of the Royal College of Physicians Edinburgh*, 27 (Supplement 3), 1997:1-11.

Pope, Norris. "health, sanitation and housing: in Schlicke (1999) 469-474.

Porter, Dorothy. "Public Health." In: Bynum and Porter (1993).

Porter, Roy and Rousseau, G.S. *Gout. The Patrician Malady*. New Haven, Yale University Press, 1998.

Porter, Roy. "Diseases of Civilization." In: Bynum and Porter (1993), 585-600.

Porter, Roy. *Disease, Medicine and Society in England 1550-1860*. London, Macmillan, 1987.

Porter, Roy. *The Greatest Benefit to Mankind*. London, Harper Collins, 1997.

Priestley, J.B. "The Great Inimitable." In: Tomlin 1969, 14-31.

Pykett, Lyn. *Charles Dickens*. Basingstoke and New York, Palgrave, 2002.

Quétel, Claude. *History of Syphilis*. Translated by Judith Braddock and Brian Pike. Baltimore, The Johns Hopkins University Press, 1990.

Radford, Edwin and Mona Augusta Radford. *Encyclopaedia of Superstitions*. Revised ed. London, Book Club Associates, 1961

Randles, Jenny and Peter Hough. Spontaneous Human Combustion. London, Hale, 1992.

Richardson, Ruth. *Death, dissection and the destitute*. London, Routledge & Kegan Paul, 1987.

Robson, W.W., "The Choir Master and the Single Buffer." In: *Critical Enquiries. Essays on Literature*. London, The Athlone Press, 1993, 139-160.

Rodin, Algin E. *Medical Literature and Eponyms: An Encyclopedia of Medical Eponyms derived from Literary Characters*. Malabar, Krieger, 1989.

Romano, John. *Dickens and Reality*. New York. Columbia University Press, 1978.

Rose, Lionel. *The massacre of the innocents. Infanticide in Britain 1988-1930*. London, Routledge and Kegan Paul, 1986.

Rosenberg, Charles E. "Medical Text and Social Context. Explaining William Buchan's *Domestic Medicine*." *Bulletin of the History of Medicine*, 57 1983:22-42.

Rothfield, Lawrence. "Medical." In: Tucker (1999),

Roulet, Ann. "A Comparative Study of *Nicholas Nickleby* and *Bleak House*." *The Dickensian* 60, 1964:117-24.

Rushdie, Salman. *Shame*. London, Cape, 1983.

"H.L.S." "Dickens and the Doctors." *St. Bartholomew's Hospital Journal*, January 1917, 43-45.

Schlicke, Paul (ed). *The Oxford Reader's Companion to Dickens*. Oxford, Oxford University Press, 1999.

Schwarzbach, F.S. "*Bleak House*: The Social Pathology of Urban Life." *Literature and Medicine* 9, 1990:93-104.

Scrimshaw, Susan C.M. "Infanticide in human populations: Societal and individual concerns." In: Hausfater, Glenn and Sarah Blaffer Hrdy, eds. *Infanticide: Comparative and Evolutionary Perspectives*. New York, Aldine Publishers, 1984, 439-462.

Seiffert, G. and Du Dscheng-Hsing. "Zur Geschichte der Pocken und Pockenimpfung." *Sudhoffs Archiv für Geschichte der Medizin und der Naturwissenschaften* 30, 1937/38:26-35.

Shaw, Sheila. "Spontaneous Combustion and the Sectioning of Female Bodies." *Literature and Medicine* 14, 1995:1-22.

Sheridan, Richard. *Plays*. London, Dent, reprint 1940.

Shore, T.H.G. "The Doctors of Dickens." *St. Bartholomew's Hospital Journal*, 1922:109-112.

Shuttleworth, Sally. *George Eliot and Victorian Science – the make-believe of a beginning.* Cambridge, Cambridge University Press, 1984.

Shryock, Richard Harrison. *The Development of Modern Medicine.* London, Knopf, 1948.

Slater, Michael. Introduction to *The Christmas Books*, London, Penguin English Library.

Small, Helen. *Love's Madness. Medicine, the Novel, and Female Insanity 1800-1865.* Oxford, Clarendon Press, 1996

Smith, Michael. "Hypnosis has real effect on pain's physiological system, study shows." *Medical Post* (Canada), March 11, 2003.

Smith, Roger. *Trial by Medicine. Insanity and Responsibility in Victorian Trials.* Edinburgh. Edinburgh University Press, 1981.

Smith, Thomas Southwood. *Use of the Dead to the Living.* Albany, 1827.

Smithers, Sir David. *Dickens's Doctors.* Oxford, Pergamon Press, 1979.

Sontag, Susan. *Illness as Metaphor.* London, Allen Lane/Penguin Books Ltd., 1979.

Spence, Gordon. Introduction to *Barnaby Rudge*. London, Penguin Classics, 1973.

Stanley, Peter. *For fear of pain. British surgery 1790-1850.* Amsterdam, Rodopi, 2003.

Stannard, Jerry. "Diseases of Western Antiquity." In: Kiple (1993), 262-270.

Storey, Graham. *Charles Dickens: Bleak House.* Cambridge, Cambridge University Press, 1987.

Summers, Anne. "The Costs and Benefits of Caring. Nursing and Charities 1830-1960." In: Barry and Jones (1991), 133-148

Tambling, Jeremy. "Death and Modernity in *Dombey and Son.*" *EIC* 43, 1993:308-329.

Temkin, Owsei. *The Falling Sickness A History of Epilepsy from the Greeks to the Beginnings of Modern Neurology.* 2nd ed, revised. Baltimore, Johns Hopkins Press, 1971.

Thackeray, William Makepeace. *Vanity Fair.* Oxford, The World Classics Edition, 1983.

Tomalin, Claire. "Little Claret?" *Times Literary Supplement*, September 6, 2002, -6-7.

Tomlin, E.W.F. *Charles Dickens 1812-1870 - a centenary volume.* London, Weidenfeld and Nicolson, 1969.

Tooley, Sarah. *The History of Nursing in the British Empire.* London, S.H. Bousfield., 1906.

Tucker, H., ed. *A Companion to Victorian Literature and Culture.* Malden, MA, Blackwell, 1999.

Tytler, Graeme. *Physiognomy in the European Novel. Faces and Fortunes.* Princeton, Princeton University Press, 1982.

Umber, George. "Dickens's Doctors." Comedy. *Kilmornock Standard,* June 22, 1912.

Valverde, Mariane. "The Love of Finery: Fashion and the Fallen Woman in Nineteenth Century Social Discourse." *Victorian Studies* 32, 1989:169-188.

Vogt, Irmgard. “Alkoholkonsum. Industrialisierung und Klassenkonflikte.” In: *Rausch und Realität. Drogen im Kulturvergleich*. Köln, 1981.

Von Engelhardt, Dietrich. *Medizin in der Literatur der Neuzeit.* Hürtgenwald, Pressler, 2000.

Vrettos, Athena. *Somatic Fictions. Imagining Illness in Victorian Culture.* Stanford, Stanford University Press, 1995.

Wainapel, Stanley F. “Dickens and disability.” *Disability and Rehabilitation* 18, 1996:629-632.

Walder, Dennis. *Dickens and Religion.* London, George Allen & Unwin, 1981.

Walkowitz, Judith. *Prostitution and Victorian Society. Women, Class and the State.* Cambridge, Cambridge University Press, 1980.

Ward, S.L. “Medical Practice in the Days of Charles Dickens.” *British Columbia Medical Journal 5*, 1963:521-5.

Warren, S. *The Opium Question.* London, J. Ridgway, 1840.

Weatherall, D.J. “Suppuration of the Blood: The Biology of Leukaemia, Past, Present and Future.” *Proceedings of the Royal College of Physicians Edinburgh* 27 (Supplement 3), 1997:41-49.

Webster, Charles, ed. *Caring for Health: History and Diversity.* The Open University. Health and Disease Series, Book 6. The Open University Press, reprint 1995.

West, John B. “Krook’s Death by Spontaneous Combustion and the controversy between Dickens and Lewes: A Physiologist’s View.” *The Dickensian* 90, 1994:125-129.

Whipple, Edwin Percy. *Charles Dickens. The Man and His Work* in two volumes. Boston and New York, Houghton Mifflin Company, 1912.

Wilks, Samuel. “Indiscriminate Use of Alcoholic Stimulants in Disease.” *The Lancet.* 1867:505-7.

Wilson, Leonard G. “Fevers.” In: Bynum and Porter (1992), 382-411.

Winnifrith, Tom. *Fallen Women in the Nineteenth Century Novel.* Basingstoke, Macmillan, 1994.

Winslow, Joan. “*The Old Curiosity Shop* – the meaning of Nell’s Fate. *The Dickensian* 88, 1981: 162-167.

Winter, Alison. *Mesmerised: powers of mind in Victorian Britain.* Chicago, University of Chicago Press, 1998.

Wolf, Peter. “Epilepsy in Literature.” *Epilepsia*, 36 (Suppl. 2) 1995:S12-S19.

Wood, Jane. *Passion and Pathology in Victorian Fiction.* Oxford, Oxford University Press, 2001.

Woods, Matthew. *In Spite of Epilepsy*. New York, The Cosmopolitan Press, 1913.

Woodward, J. and Richards, D (eds). *Health Care and Popular Medicine in Nineteenth-Century England.* London, Croom Helm, 1977.

Young, R.T. “Doctors and Diseases in Dickens.” *Cornhill Magazine* June 1934, 709.

Appendix 1 Dickens's Medical Practitioners

1. ***Sketches by Boz*** (1836)

"Four Sisters"

Mr. Dawson	Surgeon attending Mrs. Robinson's confinement
	monthly nurse assisting Mr Dawson

"Boarding House"

Dr Wosky	Mrs. Bloss's physician
Septimus Hicks	Medical student

"The Hospital Patient"
house surgeon
dressers

"The Black Veil"
nameless surgeon

"The very friendly young gentleman"
Mr Mincin

"The Mudfog and Other Sketches" 1837
First meeting
- Mr. Knight Bell
- Dr W. R. Fee
- Dr Kutankumagen (of Moscow)
- Professor Muff
- Dr Neeshawts
- Professor Nogo
- Dr Toorell

Second meeting
- Dr Grummidge
- Mortair
- Pessell
- Mr. Pipkin (M.R.C.S.)
- Dr Soemup

2. ***Pickwick Papers*** (1837)

Bob Sawyer	Medical student later doctor in Bristol and Bengal
Benjamin Allen	Medical student and doctor and friend of Bob Sawyer
Gunter	Medical Student
Noddy	Medical student
Jack Hopkins	Medical student
nameless	Medical student "pale youth with a plaited watchguard"
nameless	Medical student: "prim personage in clean linen and cloth boots"
Nockemorf	Bob Sawyer's predecessor in practice in Bristol
Slasher	Eminent surgeon at Saint Bartholomew's Hospital
Dr Payne	Military surgeon of the 43rd
Dr Slammer	Military surgeon of the 97th
nameless	treats Tupman's wound
nameless	in attendance on the pregnant Mrs Trundle
nameless	called in to attend Mrs Weller in her final illness

3. ***Oliver Twist*** (1838)

Nameless	Parish surgeon at workhouse
Parish apothecary's apprentice	called when the pauper woman, Sally, is dying
Mr. Losberne	Doctor to Mrs. Maylie and Rose Fleming
nameless	at Mr. Brownlow's
nameless	surgeon who lives near Grimwig
nameless	treats Rose Maylie in Losberne's absence.

4. ***Nicholas Nickleby***, (1839)

Dr Lumbey	Doctor attending Mrs. Kenwig's confinement
Sir Tumley Snuffim	Mrs. Wititterly's doctor
nameless	treats Smike, Madelaine Bray (same man?)

5 ***The Old Curiosity Shop*** (1841)

nameless	called in to treat grandfather
nameless	Doctor who treats Nell at the inn
nameless	treats Dick Swiveller
(The Marchioness	as nurse)

6. ***Barnaby Rudge*** (1841)

nameless surgeon	treats Haredale
nameless doctors	all agree that John Willet should die after his stroke

7. ***American Notes*** (1842)

There are several doctors, but since they are not figures of Dickens's creating, they are not listed here.

8. ***Martin Chuzzlewit***, (1844)

Bevan (USA)	seldom or never practised
Dr Ginery Dunkle	Spokesman at the Program levee, not certainly medical
John Jobling	Anthony Chuzzlewit's doctor
	Also medical office to the Anglo-Bengalee insurance company.
Lewsome	Medical assistant supplying poison to Jonas Chuzzlewit
apothecary	called in to treat Old Martin
nameless	treats Lewsome at inn

(Sairey Gamp, Betsey Prig as nurses)

9. ***Dombey & Son*** (1848)

Sir Parker Peps	Court physician present at Paul Dombey's birth and death
Pilkins	Mr. Dombey's family doctor
apothecary	called in for Paul in Brighton
surgeons	treat Dombey after fall from horse
nameless	treat Mrs Skewton

(Mrs Blockitt, Mrs Wickham as nurses)

10 ***The Christmas Books***

The Battle of Life (1846)

Alfred Heathfield	Ward of the philosopher Dr Anthony Jeddler

11 ***David Copperfield*** (1850)

Mr. Chillip	Doctor attending Mrs. Copperfield at David's birth
nameless	attend Dora, Mrs Steerforth

(nurse at David's birth)

12. ***Bleak House*** (1853)

nameless Scot	called in when Nemo dies
nameless	attends Esther and Charley
Bayham Badger	Doctor in Chelsea, trained Woodcourt
Allan Woodcourt	Takes position as Poor Law doctor
Harold Skimpole	Protégé of John Jarndyce; doesn't practice
Richard Carstone	student, would-be "M.R.C.S."

13. ***Little Dorrit*** (1857)

Dr Haggage	Marshalsea prisoner attending the birth of Amy Dorrit
Physician	Doctor to Mr. Merdle, an experienced and wise practitioner
surgeon at Bart's	treats Cavelletto

14 ***Hard Times*** (1854)

nameless — called in to attend Mrs Blackpool; probably same man called in after Steven is found in the mine.

(Sissy Jupe/Rachael as nurses)

15. **"The Lazy Tour of Two Idle Apprentices"** (1857)

(with Wilkie Collins)

Dr Speddie — Treats Thomas Idle's sprained ankle

Dr Lorn — Assistant to Speddie

(not entirely fictitious)

16. ***Reprinted Pieces*** (1858)

"Our Bore"

Callow, Clatter, Jilkens,

Snugglewood — A set of doctors making diagnoses and giving prescriptions

"Detective Police"

Dr Dundey — Robbed a bank, apprehended in America, not certainly medical

17. ***A Tale of Two Cities*** (1859)

Alexander Manette — Lucie's father, 18 years in the Bastille; more important as patient

18 ***The Uncommercial Traveller*** (1860)

"Dullborough Town"

Joe Specks — old classmate of the "Uncommercial" (possibly not entirely fictitious)

19. ***Great Expectations*** (1861)

nameless — called to attend Mrs Joe

(Biddy, Joe, Herbert as nurses)

20. ***Our Mutual Friend*** (1865)

nameless — treats Riderhood after near drowning

nameless — treat Eugene after Bradley's attack

(Jenny, Liz as nurses)

21 ***Christmas Stories*** (1867)

"No Thoroughfare" (with Wilkie Collins)

Dr Ganz	Physician in Neuchâtel

"Mrs. Lirriper's Legacy"

Dr Joshua Lirriper	Younger brother of Mrs. Lirriper's late husband.

22. ***The Mystery of Edwin Drood*** (1870)

(only in a fragment found in manuscript)

Peartree	M.R.C.S. and Member of the Eight Club

Appendix 2 Glossary

Achondroplasia	The most common and best-known form of short-limbed, short stature dwarfism.
Acute lymphocytic leukaemia	The most common form of childhood leukaemia
Anamnesis	The patient's "case history", which should include both medical and personal information.
Anorexia (adj: anorexic)	Organic or functional lack of appetite in puberty, most common as *A. nervosa,* in which particularly young girls refuse to eat for fear of becoming overweight.
Apnea	Respiratory arrest.
Argyll-Robertson pupil	(Douglas Argyll-Robertson, 1837-1909, Scottish physician) immobile, narrow pupil with maintained convergence reaction.
Ataxia	Inability to coordinate voluntary muscular movements.
Atherothromboembolic disease	A disease in which blood clots impede the flow of blood in the blood vessels.
Cerebral ischaemia	Impaired blood supply to the brain.
Clubfoot	A congenital deformity of the foot which may take several forms; early correction is possible in many cases.
Coeliac disease (non-tropical sprue)	A chronic nutritional disturbance (identified in 1936) in which the protein gluten and certain fats cannot be digested and utilized.
Contraindicated	Improper or undesirable as treatment in the given situation
Coxalgia	Pain in the the hip joint.
Coxitis	Inflammatory disease of the hip joint, due, among other things, possibly to tuberculosis.
Cryotherapy	Treatment by the application of cold.
Diencephalic syndrome	A malfunction syndrome of the diencephalon (posterior part of the forebrain) with a variety of causes, such as tumour or bleeding; first signs include behavioural changes and reduced vigilance.
Dropsy	Fluid retention with swelling of tissues.
Dysgraphia	Inability to write.
Dysphasia	Attention disorder with speech impairment.
Dyspnea	Any form of impaired breathing
Emphysema	Condition of the lung marked by abnormal dilation of airspaces and distention of lung wall; often with impaired heart function.
Enteric disorders	Disorders of the intestines.
Epilepsy	Disorder characterised by disturbed electrical rhythms of the central nervous system.

Epistaxis	Nosebleed.
Erysipelas	Streptococcus inflammation of the skin.
Distal	Further away from the point of reference; opposite is proximal
Focal dystonia	Localized abnormal muscle tone.
Foetal alcohol syndrome	Alcohol-related damage to the unborn child; characteristic are small upper lip, wide space between lip and nose, flattened bridge of nose, stubby fingers, mental retardation with increased aggression.
Gout	*Arthritis urica.* Metabolic disorder characterised by attacks of painful joint inflammation and high levels of uric acid in the blood.
Hectic fever	A fluctuating but persistent fever [from the Greek *hektikos*; habitual, consumptive – *Webster*].
Hemiplegia	Paralysis of one side of the body.
Hodgkin's Disease	(Thomas Hodgkin, 1798 – 1866, English physician) A form of cancer arising to 90% in lymph nodes.
Hypersomnia	Excessive sleepiness.
Ischaemia	Localized anemia due to interrupted blood flow.
Jargon aphasia	Inability to articulate, speech pattern of neologisms incomprehensible to the listener.
Kleine-Levin Syndrome	(Willi Kleine, 20th C German psychiatrist and Max Levin, *1901, US neurologist) Syndrome in late puberty with episodic sleeplessness and somnolence, glandular impairments resulting in overeating, weight gain (or lack of appetite and weight loss), increased (or decreased) libido.
Locomotor ataxia	*tabes dorsalis*, or neurosyphilis affecting the posterior spinal column. Slow onset with later unsteadiness of gait.
Lymphadenopathy	See Hodgkin's disease; etiology unclear, fatal if untreated.
Lymphoma	Enlargement of lymph nodes of various causes and designations: malignant lymphoma = lymphatic leukaemia.
Malaria	A protozoan disease transmitted to humans by the bite of the *Anopheles* mosquito, characterised by alternating peaks of fever and troughs of normal or low temperature.
Marfan Syndrome	(Jean Bernard Antoine Marfan, 1858-1942, French paediatrician) An inherited, generalized disorder of connective tissue with ocular, skeletal and cardiovascular manifestations. Both Abraham Lincoln and Charles deGaulle are considered possible Marfan victims.

Menière's Disease	(Prosper Menière, French neurologist, 1799-1862). Neurological disease involving, among other things, severe dizziness.
Miasma	A vapourous exhalation of rotting matter, thought to cause disease.
Myalgia	Pain in one or more muscles.
Neonate	Newborn
Paget's Disease of Bone	(Sir James Paget, 1814 – 1899, English surgeon and pathologist). Chronic skeletal disease. In one of its forms, there is characteristic bowing of the thighbone.
Paraplegia	Paralysis of both lower limbs due to injury or disease.
Parkinson's Disease	"Shaking palsy" described in 1817 by James Parkinson (1755-1824).
per os	by mouth; oral application of medication
Perthes'-Disease	Perthes-Calvé Disease (Georg Perthes, 1869-1927, German surgeon; Jacques Calvé 1875-1954, French orthopedist) Hip deformity of childhood.
Phenylalanine	Water-soluble amino acid, which is essential to the nutrition of humans and animals.
Phenylketonuria	Inborn error of metabolism, frequently resulting in mental retardation.
Phthisis	Consumption, especially *phthisis pulmonum*, or pulmonary tuberculosis.
Phythotherapeutics	Medications having active ingredients obtained from plants.
pia mater	A thin vascular membrane that invests the brain and spinal cord internal to the arachnoid (thin membrane between the pia mater and dura mater) and dura mater (tough membrane surrounding the brain).
Podagra	Gout.
Pott's Disease	(Percival Pott, English surgeon, 1713-1788). Tubercular inflammation of the spinal column.
Prodrome	A symptom/symptoms indicating the onset of disease
Purpura	Skin reddening due to bleeding below the skin.
Renal colic	Urinary tract obstruction with excruciating pain.
Renal tubular acidosis	Chronic metabolic hyperacidity resulting in muscle weakness and paralysis among other things; associated loss of bone calcium results in rickets.
Rickets (adj: rachitic)	Vitamin D deficiency due to inadequate supply, abnormal metabolism or resistance of the tissues to its action.
Scoliosis	Curvature of the spine.
Scrofula	Tuberculosis of the lymph nodes.

Scurvy	Vitamin C deficiency. In childhood, bleeding into the membrane of connective tissue of long bones causes painful swelling. Other hemorrhages may result in death if the disease is left untreated.
Syndrome	A group of signs and symptoms which occur together and characterize an abnormal state.
Torticollis	Condition in which the neck is twisted and the head inclined to one side, caused by spasmodic contractions of the neck muscles. Also called wry neck; may be psychosomatic.
Tourette's Syndrome	Georges Gilles de la Tourette, French physician, 1857-1904). Multiple compulsive tics (movements) with compulsive utterance of vile words.
Tracheobronchial tree	The ramification (branched configuration) of airways.
Typhoid Fever	General infection characterized by continuous fever, slowed heart beat, rose-colored eruption. The source is the feces of carriers. In communities with poor sanitation, transmission is most frequently by water, next by food, especially milk. This is what was usually meant when "fever" was said by laymen.
Typhus	Acute, often severe disease characterized by prolonged high fever, headache and rash. Transmitted by lice.
Uremia	In current usage, the signs and symptoms of chronic renal failure
Vesicles	A small skin elevation usually containing a clear fluid
Wry neck	See Torticollis.

Appendix 3 Medical/Medicine-related Books in Dickens's Library

There are two known lists of books in Dickens's personal library; the first at Devonshire Terrace, where he lived from December 1839 to November 1851 and the second at Gads Hill, where he lived from March 1856 to his death in 1870.

The list from Devonshire Terrace is printed in the Pilgrim edition of the *Letters*, Volume 4, Appendix C: Inventory of Contents of 1 Devonshire Terrace, May 1844. Inventory of the books (p 711-25). The Gads' Hill list is reprinted from Sotheran's "Price Current of Literature", Nos. CLXXV and CLXXVI: "Catalogue of the Library of Charles Dickens from Gadshill".

There are many books listed on travel, natural history, history and supernatural reports in addition to the medical/medicine-related texts excerpted here.

<u>Devonshire Terrace</u>

Waterton's Essay on Natural History, Charles Waterton, 1838

Dodd's Reflections on Death (1769)

Anatomy of Drunkenness [Dr Robert Macnish, 1827]

Burton's Anatomy of Melancholy (1837)

Pursuit of Knowledge under Difficulties, 1830/31; G.L.Craik

Townshend's Mesmerism [Chauncy Hare Townshend, Facts in Mesmerism, 1840]

Pettigrew's Medical Superstitions, [T.J. Pettigrew, 1844]

Management of the Poor in Scotland [W.P. Alison, Observations on the…, 1840]

Dr Robert Macnish, Philosophy of Sleep, 1840

Charities of London; S. Low and John Brownlow A Pocket Guide to the.., 1836]

Gads Hill

Most of the books in Devonshire Terrace collection, plus writings of other novelists, his own in various languages, essays on a wide variety of topics and the following:

Bell, (Sir C.)	*Anatomy and Philosophy of Expression* (1847)
Brande (Prof.)	*Dictionary of Science, Literature and Art, comprising the History, Description and Scientific Principles of every Branch of Human Knowledge* (1852)
Browne (Sir T.)	*ReligioMedici; and Hydrotophia or Urn-Burial; a Discourse on Sepulchral Urns with preliminary Discourse and Notes by J.A. St. John* (1838)
Chalmers (Dr)	Bridgewater Treatise on the *Adaptation of External Natural to the Moral and Intellectual Constitution of Man* (1853)
Conolly (Dr)	Croonian Lectures delivered at the Royal College of Physicians, 1849: "On some of the Forms of Insanity"
Cooper (S. Surgeon)	*Dictionary of Practical Surgery, comprehending the most interesting Improvements from the earliest times, the Instruments and Remedies, Etymology and Signification of Terms, etc.* (1838)
Darwin (C)	*Origin of the Species* (1860)
Dixon (Hepworth), John Howard	*London Prisons, with Account of the more Distinguished Prisoners; and a Description of the Chief Provincial Prisons* (1850)
Elliotson (Dr)	*Human Physiology; with which is incorporated part of Blumenbach's Institutiones Physicae.* (1840)
Ferrier (Prof)	*Institutes of Metaphysic; The Theory of Knowing and Being* (1854)
Harrison (JB, Surgeon)	*Medical Aspects of Death, and the Medical Aspects of the Human Mind.* (1852)
Hollingshead (John)	*Underground London, a series of Essays.* (1862
Hood (Dr WC)	*Statistics of Insanity – embracing a Report of the Bethleham Hospital 1846-1859* (1862)
Hood (Dr WC)	*Suggestions for the future Provision of Criminal Lunatics* (1854)

Hooper (Dr R)	*Medical Dictionary; of the Terms in Human and Comparative Anatomy, Botany, Chemistry, Forensic Medicine, Materia Medica, Obstetrics, Pharmacy, Physiology, Practice of Physic, Surgery, Toxicology etc.* (1848)
Jung-Stilling	*Theory of Pneumatology in reply to the question, What ought to be believed or disbelieved concerning Presentiments, Visions, and Apparitions.* (Translated by Jackson) (1854)
Lewes (GH)	*Physiology of Common Life.* 2 volumes (1859)
Macnish (Dr R)	*Philosophy of Drunkenness* (1840)
Morley (Henry)	*Life of Girolamo Cardano of Milan, Physician* (1854)
Pettigrew (TJ)	*History of Mummies* (1834)
Stallard (JH)	*London Pauperism ... Out-door Relief* (1867)
Townshend (CH)	*Mesmerism proved True and the Quarterly Reviewer reviewed* (1834)

In addition to the books, Dickens owned a number of pamphlets on various topics, including the following:

Plea for Ragged Schools

Remarks on Medical Organization and Reform

5 pamphlets on anaesthetics by J.Y. Simpson

Elliotson on a number of cases of Surgical Operations without Pain in the Mesmeric State

Abstracts of "Researches on magnetism and on Certain Allied Subjects"
(Baron von Reichenbach, abridged by Dr. W. Gregory)

The Incubation of Insanity by Forbes Winslow

Sir W. Clay's Remarks on the Water Supply of London

Walker's Lectures on the Condition of Metropolitan Graveyards (4 series)

"Healthy Homes" by Prof. Hosking

Temperance and Total Abstinence by Spencer Thomson

Report on a general Scheme for Extramural Sepulture (1850)

The General Malaria of London

Observations on London Milk by H. Rug

Urban Burial by J.D. Parry (1847)

Sanitary Requirements of the City of London by Dr J. Duke (1846)

Pictures of Pauperism (Glasgow 1847)

Children employed in Calico Print Works (1845)

Physical and Moral Condition of Children and Young Persons employed in Mines and Manufactures (1843)

Appendix 4 Related Articles and Speeches

This appendix offers an overview of the speeches given by Dickens and articles published in *Household Words* or *All the Year Round* (with the author's name, where known) which are related to the chapters in this dissertation. As might be expected, the majority of the articles deal with public health issues. The list is selective and does not include many articles published on scientific topics, even those related to medicine, such as how bones are formed or the function of the skin or lungs. The reader is referred to Anne Lohrli's *Household Words* and Ella Oppenlander's *All the Year Round* indices. There is also extensive correspondence on record between Dickens and men like Dr Southwood Smith and Henry Austin, especially on topics relevant to public health issues.

Sources:	HW/*Household Words*, *AYR*/*All the Year Round*, *Speeches* in the collection by K.J. Fielding. *The Uncommercial Traveller* (UT)
Authors:	The following authors are included; some names are abbreviated as given in the list. [information taken from Lohrli for *HW* and Oppenlander for *AYR*].

Cape	Possibly George A. Cape, Jr. Secretary to the Lambeth Baths and Wash Houses Co.
Carter, Robert Brudenell	Surgeon, studied at London Hospital. MRCS; FRCS
Dickens	CD
Dixon, Edmund Saul	Theologian and writer
Dodd, George	Writer
Hollingshead, John	Journalist, theatre manager
Horne, Richard Henry	Journalist (RHH)
Hunt, Frederick Knight	Studied medicine at Middlesex Hospital, MRCS. (FKH)
Jerdan, William	Journalist
Jerrold, William Blanchard	Journalist and author (WBJ)
Knox, James	Possibly Edinburgh publisher (Sutherland and Knox)
Leigh, Percival	Studied medicine at St. Bartholomew's Hospital. MRCS
Lewis, John Delaware	Writer
Linton (or **Lynn**), Eliza	Journalist and novelist (ELL)
MacAdam	not identified
Macpherson, Ossian	not identified
Martineau, Harriet	Writer
Morley, Henry	tudied medicine at King's College, London. (HM)
Ollier, Edmund	Poet, son of Leigh Hunt's publisher
Parkinson, Joseph Charles	Writer (JCP)
Parry, John Docwra	Clergyman
Priestley, Sir William O.	Physician, assistant to James Young Simpson in Edinburgh before moving to London
Proctor, Adelaide Anne	Daughter of BW Proctor
Proctor, Bryan Waller	London solicitor, Commissioner of Lunacy 1832-61
Sala, George Augustus	Journalist (GAS)
Smales	Not identified
Stone, Dr. Thomas	Studied medicine in Edinburgh
Strange, Charles	Chemist and druggist
Thornbury, George Walter	Artist, turned to writing

Thomas, R.M.	Not identified
Tiffin	Not identified
White, James	Churchman
Wills, William Henry	Assistant Editor; contributed earlier to *Punch* and *Bentley's Miscellany.* (WHW)
Wilson,, Florence	Governess to a "noble family at St. Petersburg during the Crimean War"
Wynter, Andrew	Physician; studied at St. George's Hospital, London and University of St. Andrews. MRCP

Chap.	Source Vol./Page	Date m/d/y	Author	Title	Topic
1	***HW*** II/137	11/2/**50**	FKH	A Great Day for Doctors	Medical school
	III/576	9/6/**51**	CD	Supposing	Prisoners vs. paupers
	IX 588	8/5/**54**	GAS	The Faculty	Medical men
	X/217	10/21/54	HM	Medical Practice Among the Poor	
	XIV/108	8/16/**56**	HM	Apothecaries	
	XVI/25	7/11/**57**	HM	Doctors' Bills	Parliament + medical profession
	AYR I/20	4/30/**59**	B.W. Proctor?	The Workhouse Nurse (verse)	
	I/416	8/27/59	HM	Buying a Practice	Problems of a newly-qualified doctor
	II/206	12/24/59	CD	Leigh Hunt, A Remonstrance	[see Skimpole]
	II/537	3/21/**60**		Bedside Experiments	Nursing
	II/566	4/7/60		Paying the Doctor	Recommends a sort of health insurance
	VIII/380	12/27/**62**	HM	The Modern Alchemist	Dr. A.S. Taylor at Guy's Hospital
	XVIII/255	9/7/**67**		Licensed to Kill	Inexperienced, unqualified doctors
2	***HW*** III/13	3/29/**51**	PL	The Rational Doctors	Nature and treatment of disease
	VII/179	5/10/51	PL	Some Account of Chloroform	
	VI/427	1/15/**53**	HM	Information against a poisoner	Malaria
	VII/421	7/2/53	Dodd	Books for the Blind	
	VIII/255	11/12/53	Knox and WHW	Colour-Blindness	
	VIII/348	12/10/53	Cape	Miasma (verse)	
	VIII/524	1/28/**54**	HM	Chip: Your Very Good Health	Dr Southwood Smith
	IX/134	3/25/54	H. Martineau	Deaf Mutes	
	IX/317	5/20/54	H. Martineau	Three Graces of Christian Science	Teaching disabled children
	IX/421	6/17/54	H. Martineau	Blindness	

Chap	Source Vol./Page	Date m/d/y	Author	Title	Topic
2, cont.	***HW*** XIV/464	11/29/**56**	Dixon	Psellism	Stammering
	XV/23	1/3/**57**	HM	A Few Really Great Men	Giants
	XIX/321	3/5/**59**	HM	At Work in the Dark	London workshop for the blind
3	***AYR*** I/36	5/7/**59**		Trade Songs: The Crossing Sweep (verse)	
	II/392	2/18/**60**	CD (UT)	Wapping Workhouse	Includes epilepsy ward
	IV/210	12/8/60		Poor Law Doctors	Includes vaccination as duty of the doctor
6	***AYR*** XIII/376	5/13/**65**		Circumlocutiona l Vaccination	Compulsory Vaccination Bill revision
7	***HW*** 1/43	4/6/**50**	George Hogarth + WHW	Heathen and Christian Burials	Needed burial reforms
	I/49	4/3/50	WHW	The Troubled Water Question	London water supply
	I/96	4/20/50	CD	Supposing	Needed reforms
	I/121	5/4/50	CD + WHW	The Heart of Mid-London	Smithfield Market
	I/186	5/18/50	HM	Letter from a Highly Respectable Old Lady	Sanitation, health
	I/301	6/22/50	P Leigh	Address from an Undertaker to the Trade	
	I/325	6/29/50	RHH	Cattle-Road to Ruin	London Slaughterhouses
	I/330	6/29/50	FKH	The Registrar General on "Life" in London	Mortality statistics
	I/361	7/13/50	Taylor + WHW	A Day in a Pauper Palace	Institution for pauper children at Swinton
	I/377	7/13/50	WHW	Chips: from Mr Thomas Bovington	Relocation of Smithfield Market
	I/451	8/3/50	WHW	Lungs for London	Proposed park in Finsbury

Chap	Source Vol./Page	Date m/d/y	Author	Title	Topic
7, cont.	*HW* I/460	8/10/50	WHW	Health by Act of Parliament	
	I/482	8/17/50	HM	The Water-Drops: A Fairy-Tale	Water pollution
	I/517	8/24/50	WHW	Chip: No Hospital for Incurables	
	II/145	10/12/50	RHH	The Cow with the Iron Tail	Adulteration of milk
	II/155	10/12/50	WHW	Poison Sold Here!	Nonrestricted sale of arsenic
	II/217	11/30/50	CD	Mr Booley's View of the Last Lord Mayor's Show	Sanitation Reform
	II/265	12/14/50	CD	A December Vision	Responsibility for righting social wrongs
	II/277	12/14/50	Strange + WHW	Death in the Teapot	Deleterious substances in tea
	II/277	12/14/50	Lewis	City Graves (verse)	
	II/323	12/28/50	Strange + WHW	Death in the Breadbasket	Deleterious substances in bread
	II/337	1/4/**51**	CD	The Last Words of the Old Year	Needed reforms
	II/413	1/25/51	Stone	The Physiology of Intemperance	
	II/426	1/25/51	WHW	Death in the Sugar Plum	Poisons in sweetmeats
	II/445	2/1/51	RHH	Father Thames	Polluted water
	II/457	2/8/51	FKH	Twenty-four Hours in a London Hospital	
	II/553	3/8/51	CD	A Monument of French Folly	Well-managed cattle market and abattoir
	II/562	3/8/51	T.M. Thomas	A Suburban Connemara	Squalid London district
	II/572	3/8/51	Macphers on	The Smithfield Model of the Model Smithfield	Cattle market
	III/25	4/5/51	CD + WHW	Spitalfields	

Chap	Source Vol./Page	Date m/d/y	Author	Title	Topic
7, cont.	HW III/193	5/24/**51**	R.H. Horne	The Pen and the Pickaxe	Sewerage drainage of outlying London districts
	III/204	5/24/51	HM	The World of Water	
	III/505	8/25/51	CD	Whole Hogs	Fanatic advocacy of temperance, etc.
	IV/145	8/1/511	CD	Sucking Pigs	Bloomerism, women with "a mission"
	IV/277	12/13/51	R. Horne	Household Crime	Arsenic poisoning
	V/31	3/27/**52**	Tiffin	King Dirt. A Song adapted to a Slow Sanitary Movement (Verse)	
	V45	4/3/52	CD + HM	Drooping Buds	Hospital for Sick Children
	V/77	4/10/52	A. Wynter	St. George and the Dragon	St. George's Hospital
	V/152	5/1/52	HM	One of the Evils of Match-Making	Phosphorus disease
	V/422	7/17/52	WHW	Mr Bovington on the new Cattle Market	Proposed site
	V/423	7/17/52	HM	Constitutional Trials	Food adulteration
	VI/97	10/16/52	G. Dodd	Penny Wisdom	Utilization of refuse and waste products
	VI/275	12/4/52	HM	Another Lung for London	Plan for model living and working community
	VI/289	12/11/52	HM	A Foe Underfoot	London's sewers
	VI/496	2/5/**53**	WHW	Clean Water and Dirty Water	Sewage disposal and water supply
	VII/49	3/19/53	CD + WHW	Received a Blank Child	Foundling Hospital
	VII/107	4/2/53	HM	Fresh Air in Finsbury	Proposed park
	VII/169	4/12/53	CD	Home for Homeless Women	Urania Cottage
	VII/179	4/23/53	HM	Chloroform	
	VII/234	5/7/53	HM	A Puff of Smoke	Tobacco smoking

Chap	Source Vol./Page	Date m/d/y	Author	Title	Topic
7, cont.	***HW*** VII/601	8/27/**53**	G. Sala	Want Places	Female Servants
	VIII/97	10/1/53	CD	Frauds on the Fairies	Misappropriation of fairy-tales for teetotalism
	VIII/156	10/15/53	G. Sala	More Places Wanted	Female Servants
	VIII/169	10/22/53	HM	The Modern Practice of Physic	
	VIII/524	1/28/**54**	HM	Your Very Good Health	Summary of sanitary improvements
	VIII/575	2/11/54	WBJ	The Iron Seamstress	Sewing machines
	IX/158	4/1/54	ELL	The Rights and Wrongs of Women	
	IX/257	4/29/54	ELL	One of our Legal Fictions	19th C English laws for women
	IX/398	6/10/54	HM	Death's Doors	Dwellings of the poor
	IX/447	6/24/54	HM	The War with Fever	Operation of common lodging houses
	IX/464	7/1/54	?	Smoke or No Smoke	Smoke nuisance in London
	X/196	10/14/54	HM	Piping Days	London sewerage
	X/276	11/4/54	Smales	The Moral of This Year (Verse)	Epidemics of 1854
	X/292	11/11 /54	HM	A Home Question	Public health
	X/319	11/18/54	HM	Commission and Omission	London drainage and sewerage
	X/409	12/16/54	HM	Conversion of a Heathen Court	Renovation of London tenements
	X/560	1/27/**55**	A Proctor	Cradle Song of the Poor (verse)	
	XI/193	3/31/55	HM	Frost-bitten Homes	Poor in Bethnal Green
	XI/213	3/31/55	HM	Starvation of an Alderman	Hassall's "Food and its Adulteration" [*Lancet*]
	XII/85	8/25/55	HM	Wild Court Tamed	Renovation of tenements
	XII/265	10/20/55	HM	An Enemy's Charge	Intramural burials
	XII/457	12/15/55	HM	Hospitals	

Chap.	Source Vol./Page	Date m/d/y	Author	Title	Topic
7, cont.	***HW*** XIII/25	1/26/**56**	CD	A Nightly Scene in London	The shelterless poor
	XIII/121	2/23/56	G. Sala	Houseless and Hungry	London refuge for the destitute
	XIII/220	3/22/56	HM	Poison	
	XIII/397	5/10/56	ELL	Epidemics	Review of Southwood Smith's book
	XIII/420	5/17/56	Harvey	Strychnine	
	XIV/313	10/18/56	R.B. Carter	Health and Education	Young ladies' schools
	XV/234	3/7/**57**	HM	Many Needles in one Housewife	Lodgings for working girls
	XVI/193	8/29/57	HM	A Healthy Year in London	Medical Officer's reports
	XVI/226	9/5/57	HM	Burning, and Burying	Report on cremation by a surgeon (MRCS)
	XVI/333	10/3/57	HM	Lord W. Tyler	Legislation on lodgings for the poor
	XVI/564	12/17/57	HM	A Piece of Work	Dr Roth's recommendations for gymnastics etc
	XVII/73	1/9/**58**	HM	A Lesson Lost upon Us	Sanitary measures during the Crimean War
	XVII/131	1/23/58	W. Jerdan	A British Nuisance	Animal slaughter in London
	XVII/361	4/3/58	HM	Use and Abuse of the Dead	Bodies for dissection
	XVIII/79	7/10/58	HM	A Way to Clean Rivers	Sewage disposal
	XVIII/121	7/24/58	E. Dixon	Dirty Cleanliness	Sewage disposal
	XVIII/379	10/2/58	HM	One other Hospital for Children	In Liverpool
	XVIII/433	10/23/58	E. Linton	Water	
	XIX/249	2/17/**59**	W.O. Priestley	Chloroform	
	XIX/415	4/2/59	HM	The Cure of Sick Minds	Dr Bucknill's report on lunatic asylums
	XIX/546	5/7/59	F. Wilson	Only a governess	Attitudes towards governesses
	AYR I/40	5/7/**59**		A Sum in Fair Division	Poor Law and Removal Act

Chap	Source Vol./Page	Date m/d/y	Author	Title	Topic
7, cont.	***AYR*** II/74	11/19/**59**		Good Samaritans	Samaritans Free Hospital for Women and Young Children (also mentions Great Ormond St. Hospital for Sick Children
	II/506	3/24/**60**		Life in Danger	Pollution of the Serpentine
	II/530	3/31/60		Good Water	Natural rain cycle and filtering
	III/37	4/21/60	CD (UT)	The Great Tasmania's Cargo	Care of wounded soldiers being brought back from service in India
	III/85	5/5/60	CD (UT)	City of London Churches	"breathing dead parishioners" in city churches
	III/247	5/23/60		How the World Smokes	Descriptive and statistics
	III/348	7/21/60	CD (UT)	Night Walks	Houseless in London
	III/427	8/11/60		Needlewoman's Hall	Recommends a sort of union
	IV/29	10/20/60		Sanitary Science	Housing, sewerage
	IV/227	12/15/60		Registration of Sickness	Southwood Smith and Chadwick
	IV/500	3/21/**61**	J. Hollingshe ad	A New Chamber of Horrors	Satirical suggestion of Museum of Men, Women and Children who had starved to death
	IV/561	3/23/61		Magic and Science	Fresh air; superstitions
	V/44	4/6/61		Sick Pauper	Miss Elliot and Miss Cobb in Glasgow
	V/254	6/8/61		Children of all Work	Children's Employment Commission
	V/390,413,4 53,470,486	7/20/61	J. Hollings-head	Underground London	London sewers
	V/397	6/20/61	CD (UT)	The Short-timers	Half-Time system of schools (mentions Chadwick)
	V/475	8/10/61		Growth of a Hospital	London Fever Hospital
	VI/137,150	11/2/61	J. Hollings-head ?	London Water	

Chap	Source Vol./Page	Date m/d/y	Author	Title	Topic
7, cont.	***AYR*** VI/454	2/1/**62**	HM?	Between the Cradle and the Grave	London Children's Hospital
	VII/301	6/7/62	? CD + WHW	Hail Columbia-Square	Miss Coutts's housing project in Bethnal Green
	VIII/132	10/18/62		The Girl from the Workhouse	Training for girls
	VIII/232	11/15/62		The Trick of the Trapeze	Fire escapes for London tenements
	IX/188	4/18/**63**		Temperate Temperance	Real temperance harmed by intemperate advocacy
	IX/493	7/18/63	CD (UT)	The City of the Absent	City churchyards
	IX/588	8/15/63	CD (UT)	The Boiled Beef of New England	Against "Mrs Pardiggle" type of charity
	X/36	9/5/63		The Point of the Needle	Everything unchanged, despite Association for the Aid and Benefit of Dressmakers and Milliners
	X/93	9/19/63	E. Yates	Kensal Green	Cemetery
	X/205	10/24/63	CD (UT)	Titbull's Alms-Houses	Alms-houses and retreats
	XII/198	10/8/**64**		The Lives and Deaths of the People	John Simon on causes and distribution of disease
	XII/272	10/29/64		Workmen's Diseases	Scurvy, lead and mercury poisoning
	XII/326	11/12/64		Water	Scientific discussion of properties; mentioned Sydenham
	XIII/16	1/28/**65**		A Fight with Fever	London Fever Hospital
	XIII/181	3/18/65		Death in the Latest Fashions	Absurdities of Victorian burial customs
	XIII/413	5/27/65		To Smoke or Not to Smoke	Review of paper by M. Jolly, Member of the Imperial Academy of Medicine (France)
	XIII/512	6/24/65		Poverty	Especially problems of housing, sanitation

Chap	Source Vol./Page	Date m/d/y	Author	Title	Topic
7, cont.	***AYR*** XIV/176	9/16/**65**		Ill in a Workhouse	Contrasts voluntary hospitals and workhouse infirmaries (*Lancet* Commission)
	XIV/372	11/11/65	JCP	Everyman's Poison	Inspections of lodgings/*Lancet Commission*
	XIV/474	12/9/65		Village Hospitals	Need for local hospitals
	XVI/253	9/22/**66**	JCP	How Not to Do It	Condition of the Poor in England
	XVI/342	10/20/66	JCP	In Praise of a Rotten Board	Poor Law Board vs. medical advice
	XVII/221	3/2/**67**		What is Sensational ?	In response to complaint of carrying "sensational" articles about death in the workhouse. Houseless Poor Act
	XVII/282	3/16/67	G.W. Thornbury	Old Stories Retold: Resurrection Men	Burke and Hare
	XVII/352	4/6/67	JCP	Lucifer-Box Making	Child labour
	XVII/585	6/15/67	JCP	Slavery in England	Children's Employment Commission
	XVIII/541	11/30/67	JCP	A Workhouse Probe	*Lancet* Commission on Improvement of Workhouse Infirmaries
	XVIII/558	12/7/67	JCP	Another Workhouse Probe	*Lancet* Commission
	XIX/16	12/14/67	JCP	A Country Workhouse	Includes description of infirmary
	XIX, 606	6/6/**68**		Ague and its Cause	Malaria
	XX/295	9/5/68		Painless Operations	Chloroform
	XX/540	11/14/68		Canker in the Bud	Children's home in Leytonstone to "rescue tainted children from life of pollution'
	N.S.I/61	12/19/68	CD (UT)	A Small Star in the East	East London Children's Hospital

Chap	Source Vol./Page	Date m/d/y	Author	Title	Topic
7, cont.	***AYR*** N.S.I/394	3/27/**69**		Sewing Machines	Difficulties of working with the machine [*Lancet* reported the first "repetitive stress syndrome" in connection with the machine]
	N.S.II/13	6/5/69	CD	A Plea for Total Abstinence	Overloading of horses during temperance parade
	N.S.II/302	8/28/69		Little Pauper Boarders	Private boarding rather than stifling workhouse or district schools
	N.S. III/204	1/29/**70**	ELL	Getting Better	Convalescence Homes, especially those started by Mrs Gladstone
8	***HW*** IV/189	11/15/**51**	CD	Homœpathy	Review of Epp's *Principles*
	VIII/492	1/21/**54**	G. Dodd	Half-a-dozen Leeches	Odd facts about leeches
	X/97	9/16/54	E. Ollier	Faces	Physiognomy
	XI/304	4/28/**55**	MacAdam	Physic A-Field	A Rich Storehouse and Treasurie for the Diseased (16th C. treatise)
	XIII/191	3/8/**56**	HM	One Cure More	Review of Dr M. Roth's "Movement Cure"
	AYR I/497	9/17/**59**		Wonders will never cease	Superstitions (caul, etc)
	II/484	3/17/**60**		The Breath of Life	Treatments, including bleeding and opium
	V/358	7/6/**61**		Medical Nuts to Crack	Inquests; includes anecdote from Pettigrew's *Superstitions*
	VI/246	12/7/61		What Wine does for Us	Real influence of moderate wine-drinking
	VIII/519	2/7/**63**	HM?	Illiberal Doctors	Against ban on homœopathy and mesmerism in Ireland
	XIII/33	2/4/**65**		Magnesian Light	Magnesium also as antidote for gout, poison (also first electric lights)
	XIII/521	6/24/65		Wine against Physic	

Chap	Source Vol./Page	Date m/d/y	Author	Title	Topic
	AYR XVII/29	1/5/**67**		Superstition Dies Hard	Parish doctor confronted with witchcraft
	XVII/322	3/20	G.W. Thornbury	Old Stories Retold: Fieschi and the Infernal machine	Assassination attempt on Luis Philippe of France, 28. July 1835
	N.S. II/541	11/6/**69**		Witchcraft in the Nineteenth Century	
	N.S. III/9	12/4		Thermal-Water Cure	
9	***HW*** IX/61	3/4/**54**	G. Dodd + WHW	Several Heads of Hair	Traffic with and use of human hair [see Krook and Ada, *BH*]

SPEECHES

Dissertation Chapter / Page In Fielding	Speech held in	Date m/d/y	Topic
7 42	London Tavern	6/29/**43**	Dr Southwood Smith's Sanatorium
104	Freemason's Tavern, London	2/6/**50**	Metropolitan Sanitary Association
127	Gore House, Kensington	5/10/**51**	Metropolitan Sanitary Association
222	London Tavern	6/5/**56**	Royal Hospital for Incurables
232	London Tavern	5/21/**57**	Royal Hospital for Incurables
246	Freemasons' Hall	2/8/**58**	Hospital for Sick Children
319	Freemasons' Tavern	5/6/**63**	Royal Free Hospital
8 65	London Tavern	4/20/**44**	Governesses' Benevolent Institution
68	London Tavern	6/4/**44**	Dr Southwood Smith's Sanatorium – talks about sick governess

Index

Entries in **bold print** refer to sections of this dissertation. Fictional characters in the works are listed separately, and **bold print** indicates sections dealing mainly with the character.

CHARACTERS

CHARACTERS from other authors